Imitators of Epileptic Seizures

C.P. Panayiotopoulos

Imitators of Epileptic Seizures

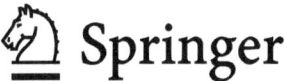 Springer

Author
C.P. Panayiotopoulos, M.D., Ph.D., F.R.C.P.
St. Thomas' Hospital
Department of Clinical Neurophysiology and Epilepsies
London
United Kingdom

ISBN 978-1-4471-4022-1   ISBN 978-1-4471-4023-8   (eBook)
DOI 10.1007/978-1-4471-4023-8
Springer Dordrecht Heidelberg New York London

Library of Congress Control Number: 2012940657

Printed on acid-free paper

Springer is part of Springer Science+Business Media (www.springer.com)

Preface

The aim of medicine is to diagnose, prevent and treat (alleviate or cure) human diseases. Accurate diagnosis is a prerequisite and the golden rule for meaningful treatment.

Imitators of epileptic seizures are a broad spectrum of episodic manifestations that mimic, "look like" but are not, epileptic seizures. They range from normal phenomena, such as hypnagogic jerks, hallucinations or illusions, to a galaxy of abnormal paroxysmal symptoms of a variety of brain and systemic disorders. Imitators of epileptic seizures occur at any age, but their highest incidence is seen in childhood, particularly during the first years of life.

Misdiagnosis of imitators of epileptic seizures as genuine epilepsy is a colossal problem affecting as many as 20–30% of patients diagnosed with, and often treated for many years for, epilepsy or admitted to tertiary care epilepsy units. The problem is complicated by the fact that approximately 30% of patients with genuine epileptic seizures also suffer from non-epileptic, mainly psychogenic, seizures.

Conversely, nearly all types of epileptic seizures can imitate non-epileptic paroxysmal events. The result is avoidable morbidity and sometimes mortality.

Distinguishing epileptic from non-epileptic disorders is fundamental to diagnosis and a classical example of differential diagnosis is the monumental book of William Richard Gowers published in 1907, *The Border-land of Epilepsy: Faints, Vagal Attacks, Vertigo, Migraine, Sleep Symptoms and their Treatment.* Today, the diagnosis of epilepsy and its imitators still relies principally on clinical history.

The clinical diagnosis is often easy and secured if individual elements of clinical events are meaningfully synthesised with regard to quantity, quality, location, onset, chronological sequence, development, speed of progress and duration. An inadequate history is the most common reason for misdiagnosis.

This concise booklet provides a physician-friendly modern review of the imitators of epileptic seizures with particular emphasis on key points of clinical significance. The aim is to assist healthcare professionals in optimising the differential diagnosis of epileptic from non-epileptic attacks and prevent misdiagnosis and incorrect treatment.

March 2012 Oxford   C.P. Panayiotopoulos, M.D., Ph.D., F.R.C.P.

Contents

Abbreviations

AED	Anti-epileptic drug
cAMP	Cyclic adenosine monophosphate
CI	Confidence interval
CNS	Central nervous system
CSF	Cerebrospinal fluid
CVS	Cyclic vomiting syndrome
ECG	Electocardiogram
EEG	Electroencephalogram
EMG	Electromyography
GTCS	Generalised tonic–clonic seizure
HLA	Human leukocyte antigen
ILAE	International League Against Epilepsy
JME	Juvenile myoclonic epilepsy
MDVU	Movement Disorders Virtual University
MRI	Magnetic resonance imaging
MSLT	Multiple sleep latency test
NEPE	Non-epileptic paroxysmal event
NREM	Non-rapid eye movement
PGTCS	Primarily generalised tonic–clonic seizure
PNEPE	Psychogenic non-epileptic paroxysmal event
RBD	REM sleep behaviour disorder
REM	Rapid eye movement
SGTCS	Secondarily generalised tonic–clonic seizure
WEMOVE	Worldwide Education and Awareness for Movement Disorders

Introduction

'Non-epileptic seizures' or 'non-epileptic paroxysmal disorders' are the currently preferred descriptive names for the common and numerous, diverse paroxysmal clinical events that mimic or look like but are not epileptic seizures.[1-3]

The ILAE[4,5] defines the imitators of epileptic seizures as:

> *Clinical manifestations presumed to be unrelated to an abnormal and excessive discharge of a set of neurons of the brain including (a) disturbances in brain function (vertigo or dizziness, syncope, sleep and movement disorders, transient global amnesia, migraine, enuresis); and (b) pseudoseizures (non-epileptic sudden behavioural episodes presumed to be of psychogenic origin; these may coexist with true epileptic seizures).*

I use the term non-epileptic paroxysmal events (NEPEs) or imitators of epileptic seizures to also include normal paroxysmal behaviours that are neither seizures nor disorders. NEPEs occur at any age, but their highest incidence is seen in childhood, particularly during the first years of life.

NEPEs misdiagnosed as epileptic seizures affect as many as 20–30% of patients diagnosed with, and often treated for many years for, epilepsy or admitted to tertiary care epilepsy units.[6-8] The problem is complicated by the fact that approximately 30% of patients with genuine epileptic seizures also suffer from non-epileptic, mainly psychogenic, seizures.

NEPEs are divided into two groups:
- Physiological or organic NEPEs
- Psychogenic NEPEs.

The physiological or organic NEPEs are a broad spectrum of episodic manifestations ranging from normal phenomena, such as hypnagogic jerks, hallucinations or illusions, to a galaxy of abnormal paroxysmal symptoms of a variety of brain and systemic disorders. The differential diagnosis is much more demanding in neonates, babies, toddlers and young children in whom there are many different causes and seizure imitators of normal and abnormal behaviours and symptoms.

The assessment of a patient referred for epilepsy should follow the same approach as any other disorder.

The clinical diagnosis is often easy and secured only if individual elements of clinical events are meaningfully synthesised with regard to quantity, quality, location, onset, chronological sequence, development, speed of progress and duration.
An inadequate history is the most common reason for misdiagnosis.

Video and video-EEG illustrations of epileptic seizures and NEPEs can be found in the CD companion of references[10-12].

Author's Note to Junior Physicians

In the process of making a diagnosis be prepared to challenge yourself with complicated cases and enrich your knowledge through the discussion of cases with other colleagues and reading about possible seizure imitators other than the epileptic disorders. The classic book by Adams and Victor, *Principles of Neurology*, now in its eight edition, is the best place to start with your reading.[9] There are also excellent and reliable website sources of information such as PubMed, WEMOVE and GeneTests. The Bookshelf of the National Center for Biotechnology Information provides free of charge a growing collection of biomedical books that can be easily searched and used (http://www.ncbi.nlm.nih.gov/sites/entrez?db=books). Amongst these books, *Imitators of Epilepsy*[3] is an excellent and relevant read. The *Merck Manuals*, a series of healthcare books for medical professionals and consumers, are now freely available in enhanced online versions (www.merck.com/mmpe/index.html); these have been appropriately updated and contain photographs, and audio and video materials.

There is always something new to learn and find. It is not shameful not to know the answer, nor is it embarrassing to ask other colleagues.

No one, even the most expert, knows everything.

Making a personal database and recording unclassified or strange cases that elude diagnosis is a very useful and rewarding learning exercise. Some of these cases may cluster either into a well-described syndrome unknown to you or constitute a new unrecognised syndrome that you may be the first to describe.

Useful Clinical Note

Diagnosis may be elusive even after the most assiduous application of clinical methods, even by astute experts.

When a definite diagnosis is not possible:

- Explain this to the patient/carers
- State it in the patient's notes
- Whenever reasonable and safe, allow time and seek additional information by clinical history, progress and tests
- Discuss or refer the patient to another colleague for a second opinion
- Avoid initiating treatment but if the paroxysmal events are potentially dangerous and epileptic seizures are the most likely diagnosis, anti-epileptic drugs (AEDs) may be started (but always be prepared to modify diagnosis and treatment).

Main Types of Epileptic Seizures and Their Imitators

Generalised Tonic–Clonic Seizures

Generalised tonic–clonic seizures (GTCSs), because of their dramatic features, are the main reason for referral for medical consultation. This first demands careful exclusion of syncope, psychogenic non-epileptic seizures and other NEPEs. Once an unequivocal diagnosis of genuine epileptic GTCS has been established, the main differential diagnosis is between primarily GTCS (PGTCS) and secondarily GTCS (SGTCS) (Table 1.1).

Considering their dramatic and stereotypical features, GTCSs should not be difficult to diagnose. So, why are NEPEs so frequently misdiagnosed as GTCSs and less often *vice versa*? There are four main reasons for this:

1. The patient is amnesic of the ictal events, although other symptoms preceding a GTCS are often of diagnostic value.

	Primarily GTCS	Secondarily GTCS
GTCS in patients who also have other clinically evident seizures	About 90%	About 90%
Typical absences	About 40%	None
Myoclonic jerks	About 60%	None
Focal seizures	None	About 90%
GTCS in patients without other clinically evident seizures[a]	About 10%	About 10%
Precipitating factors	>60%	<10%
Consistently on awakening	Common	Uncommon
Family history of similar epilepsies	Common	Uncommon
EEG in untreated patients		
Generalised discharges	About 80%	Exceptional
Focal abnormalities alone	About 10%	About 60%
Generalised discharges and focal abnormalities	About 30%	Exceptional
High-resolution brain imaging		
Focal abnormalities	Exceptional	About 60%
Normal	By definition	About 40%

[a]It is these patients, who make up about 10% of each category, that constitute the main problem in the differential diagnosis between primarily and secondarily GTCS. However, other features, such as precipitating factors, circadian distribution, EEG and brain imaging, are often of diagnostic significance

Table 1.1 Differentiation of primarily versus secondarily GTCS

C.P. Panayiotopoulos, *Imitators of Epileptic Seizures*, DOI 10.1007/978-1-4471-4023-8_1, © Springer-Verlag London 2012

2. The events have not been adequately witnessed, although the physical and mental consequences of a GTCS are often of diagnostic value.
3. The events, even when adequately witnessed and identified, are abbreviated in diagnostic terms (tonic–clonic seizures or grand mal or syncope or pseudoseizure) rather than describing in detail what had happened.
4. Previous minor paroxysmal events (which may be focal or generalised seizures) are not detected.

The medical training in GTCSs and epilepsies in general is largely inadequate (see lessons to be learned below).

That psychogenic convulsive status epilepticus can be mistaken by physicians as genuine GTCS status epilepticus – a misdiagnosis that may have avoidable and grave consequences – is of concern for all those involved.

Lessons to Be Learned

Tutorials on differential diagnosis of GTCSs

For educational purposes I often present to junior colleagues a video-recorded convulsive NEPE with a hypothetical scenario in which they witness this patient's symptoms in the accident and emergency department.

The video shows a middle-aged man who, while sitting in the company of others, slowly takes his glasses off, places them on the table and immediately smoothly slips to the floor where he stretches out, apparently unconscious and with eyes closed, hands crossed on the front of his chest and legs cycling rather than convulsing.

The attendants are allowed to see the video many times, in slow motion if they wish, before giving their diagnosis and what they are likely to put down in his medical notes. Almost all the attendants consider this a genuine GTCS, although some made the remark that this was a SGTCS in order to explain why the patient removed his glasses before the convulsions. More than 80 % would put the diagnostic term GTCS down in the patient notes, without describing the sequence of the events, although some would make a remark that there was no tongue biting or urinary incontinence. None of the attendants considered the diagnostic significance of the patient having his eyes closed during the whole event, which alone would exclude the possibility of a GTCS.[13] All attendants knew that a GTCS manifests with tonic–clonic convulsions and their sequences, but more than half had not seen a genuine GTCS, even though this should be a routine video teaching material in every medical school. The tutorial ends with the presentation and analysis of a video-recorded genuine GTCS.

Of the numerous imitators of epileptic seizures, the syncope and convulsive NEPEs are detailed in this chapter because they are the most likely of the imitators to be misdiagnosed as GTCSs. Suspicion of nocturnal GTCSs (if not witnessed by a room- or bed-partner) is usually raised by symptoms and signs that result from the direct or indirect impact of GTCSs on patients (injury, muscle pains, bedwetting, confusion), which are usually apparent when the patient wakes up.

Symptoms preceding SGTCSs have as many imitators as focal epileptic seizures.

Prodromes (Non-epileptic) Preceding the Onset of a GTCS

Prodrome is a non-epileptic, subjective or objective clinical alteration preceding the onset of an epileptic seizure by several hours. This can take the form of a headache, changes in mood or behaviour, sleep disturbances, light-headedness, anxiety and difficulty in concentrating before the attack. Prodrome should not be confused with aura, which is a brief seizure itself. Prodromes are most probably symptoms of systemic or metabolic disturbances that are the causative or precipitating factors of the following seizure (i.e. hypoglycaemia, premenstrual period). Prodromes are attributed to a pre-ictal increase of excitability of an epileptogenic focus or of the entire brain,[14] but there is no proof for this.

> *For almost all the patients whom I have seen with a diagnosis of prodrome, it was either an epileptic seizure itself (prolonged or clusters of brief, focal or generalised) or a symptom of a metabolic or electrolyte disturbance that caused the GTCS.*

The following quote was taken from a medical report of a patient with phantom absences, GTCSs and absence status epilepticus:

> *This man has GTCSs from 16 years of age. Interestingly, each of his GTCSs is preceded by a prodrome of half an hour to 12 hours of mental slowing down during which he makes some effort to formulate his response, which occasionally is inappropriate and bumbled.*

Ictal Events Preceding the Onset of a GTCS

These differ between PGTCSs and SGTCSs; for example, clusters of myoclonic jerks precede and herald PGTCSs in juvenile myoclonic epilepsy (JME), whereas SGTCSs develop from focal seizures.

Epileptic Myoclonic Jerks

There are many types of epileptic myoclonic jerks that may manifest as:
- The only manifestation of an epileptic seizure
- One component of an epileptic attack occurring in continuity with another type of seizure, such as myoclonic–atonic seizures, myoclonic absence seizures or myoclonic tonic–clonic seizures

Furthermore, in some epileptic syndromes, myoclonic jerks may be:
- The predominant, but rarely the only type of epileptic seizure
- Infrequent or inconspicuous
- Concurrent with genuine non-epileptic myoclonus or myoclonic-like jerks

Frequently, epileptic myoclonic jerks are not reported by the patient and not detected by the physicians. A typical example of this is JME.

> *The yield of detecting myoclonic jerks increases significantly by questions such as 'do you spill your morning tea easily?', 'do you become unduly clumsy in the morning?' and 'do you have sudden rigors?',*

*and mainly by physical demonstrations of what the myoclonic jerks
look like (videos may be much more useful for this).
If hypnagogic jerks are reported then it is certain that the concept
of myoclonic jerks has been understood.*

Epileptic myoclonus should be distinguished from normal myoclonic jerks, such as hypnagogic myoclonus, non-epileptic (subcortical) myoclonus and non-epileptic, non-myoclonic phenomena. Non-epileptic (subcortical) myoclonus includes:

- Essential myoclonus
- Opsoclonus–myoclonus syndrome (Kinsbourne syndrome), dancing eyes syndrome or myoclonic encephalopathy of infants; myoclonus is nearly continuous, erratic and movement-induced (action myoclonus)
- Benign neonatal sleep myoclonus
- Normal startle responses or hyperekplexia
- Psychogenic myoclonus, which is usually segmental or generalised, and usually worsens with exposure to stress or anxiety
- Toxic or drug-induced myoclonus.

Non-epileptic, non-myoclonic phenomena include:

- Tremor
- Tics
- Involuntary movements.

Diagnostic Tips

Myoclonic jerks frequently occur during any stage of sleep.

Myoclonic jerks consistently or exclusively occurring in the transitional state from wakefulness to sleep are unlikely to be epileptic.

Conversely, myoclonic jerks predominantly occurring upon awakening are probably of epileptic origin.

Absence Seizures

Absence seizures with severe impairment of consciousness should not be difficult to diagnose. However, these (including absence status epilepticus) are often misdiagnosed as NEPEs, and include episodes of daydreaming, preoccupation, mannerisms, drug-induced abnormal mental states, organic confusional states, prodromes of GTCS or transient global amnesia. NEPEs of vacant spells frequently occur in children with learning difficulties such as Rett or Lennox–Gastaut syndrome.

If there is uncertainty as to the nature of the attacks, an EEG is mandatory. A normal EEG with appropriately performed hyperventilation makes absence seizures (but not complex focal seizures) improbable.

An EEG is the most appropriate test to differentiate absence epileptic seizures from NEPEs.

Tonic Seizures

Tonic seizures of epileptic encephalopathies are sometimes inconspicuous and occur predominantly or only during sleep. Imitators of tonic seizures are NEPEs that cause sustained increase in muscle contraction such as:

- Tonic spasms of multiple sclerosis, which rarely may be a presenting symptom
- Dystonic symptoms of paroxysmal movement disorders
- Tonic reflex seizures of early infancy
- Gastro-oesophageal reflux attacks
- Occupational spasms such as writer's spasm

Epileptic Spasms

The epileptic spasms should be easy to diagnose because of the unique characteristic features of each attack and because of their serial and unprovoked clustering. However, parents and physicians often miss this.[15] Erroneous diagnoses include exaggerated startle responses or 'colic and abdominal pain', non-epileptic episodic disorders and gastro-oesophageal reflux.[15] Benign myoclonus of early infancy (Fejerman syndrome or benign non-epileptic infantile spasms)[16-18] is not an epileptic condition, but may cause diagnostic problems because of a similar age at onset and similar spasms.

Epileptic Drop Attacks

Epileptic drop attacks (synonyms: *sudden falls, astatic seizures*) are due to loss of erect posture that results from an atonic, myoclonic or tonic mechanism.[19,20] Falls may be due to atonic, myoclonic, myoclonic–atonic or tonic seizures. They are common in epileptic encephalopathies. Convulsions and loss of consciousness may not occur or may not be apparent. Falls may also occur in focal epilepsies.[21,22]

Of the imitators of epileptic astatic seizures (i.e. syncopes, movement disorders, brain-stem, otological causes like in Meniere diseases, spinal or lower limb abnormalities, cataplexy, periodic paralysis, drug-induced) the most likely to cause diagnostic problems are drop attacks associated with:

- Colloid cysts of the third ventricle
- Neurological conditions of lower limb muscle weakness with sudden give-way weakness leading to falls without impairment of awareness
- Vertebrobasilar insufficiency
- Carotid sinus hypersensitivity.

Drop attacks in the elderly are associated with high levels of morbidity; diagnoses are achievable in the majority of cases and these are unlikely to be of epileptic origin.[23]

Idiopathic drop attacks without a detectable cause manifest with sudden fall without loss of consciousness and with instantaneous recovery, although injury may occur. They are more common in middle-aged women.

Focal Epileptic Seizures

There is a myriad of normal and abnormal NEPEs that imitate focal epileptic seizures. These vary according to the type of focal epileptic seizure (Tables 1.2 and 1.3). Typical examples of NEPEs imitating focal epileptic seizures are:

- The migraine auras, déjà vu and other experiential phenomena of normal people
- Hallucinations of psychiatric patients, drug-related olfactory and other hallucinations
- Transient paraesthesias of peripheral neuropathies, paroxysmal movement disorders and parasomnias

Conversely, focal epileptic seizures may be misdiagnosed as NEPEs:

- Visual occipital seizures are commonly considered to be visual aura of migraines
- Hypermotor seizures are a typical example of mistaking epileptic seizures for NEPEs; so-called 'paroxysmal nocturnal dystonia' or 'hypnogenic paroxysmal dystonia' is frontal lobe epilepsy
- Autonomic seizures of childhood are another disturbing example of erroneous diagnoses as encephalitis, migraine, syncope, cyclic vomiting syndrome (CVS) or gastroenteritis.[24]

The differential diagnosis of focal seizures is detailed in the relevant chapters of my recent book.[23a]

Clinical seizure type	EEG seizure type	EEG inter-ictal expression
A. Simple partial seizures (consciousness not impaired)	Local contralateral discharge starting over the corresponding area of cortical representation (not always recorded on the scalp)	Local contralateral discharge
1. With motor signs		
(a) Focal motor without march		
(b) Focal motor with march (jacksonian)		
(c) Versive		
(d) Postural		
(e) Phonatory (vocalisation or arrest of speech)		
2. With somatosensory or special-sensory symptoms (simple hallucinations, e.g. tingling, light flashes, buzzing)		
(a) Somatosensory		
(b) Visual		
(c) Auditory		
(d) Olfactory		
(e) Gustatory		
(f) Vertiginous		

Table 1.2 ILAE classification of partial (focal, local) seizures

Clinical seizure type	EEG seizure type	EEG inter-ictal expression
3. With autonomic symptoms or signs (including epigastric sensation, pallor, sweating, flushing, piloerection and pupillary dilation)		
4. With psychic symptoms (disturbance of higher cerebral function). These symptoms rarely occur without impairment of consciousness and are much more commonly experienced as complex partial seizures		
(a) Dysphasic		
(b) Dysmnesic (e.g. déjà vu)		
(c) Cognitive (e.g. dreamy states, distortions of time sense)		
(d) Affective (e.g. fear, anger)		
(e) Illusions (e.g. macropsia)		
(f) Structured hallucinations (e.g. music, scenes)		
B. Complex partial seizures (with impairment of consciousness; may sometimes begin with simple symptomatology)	Unilateral or, frequently, bilateral discharge, diffuse or focal in temporal or frontotemporal regions	Unilateral or bilateral, generally asynchronous focus; usually in the temporal or frontal regions
1. Simple partial onset followed by impairment of consciousness		
(a) With simple partial features (A1 to A4) followed by impaired consciousness		
(b) With automatisms		
2. With impairment of consciousness at onset		
(a) With impairment of consciousness only		
(b) With automatisms		
C. Partial seizures evolving to secondarily generalised seizures (this may be generalised tonic–clonic, tonic or clonic) (above discharges become secondarily and rapidly generalised)		
1. Simple partial seizures (A) evolving to generalised seizure		
2. Complex partial (B) evolving to generalised seizure		
3. Simple partial seizures evolving to complex partial seizures evolving to generalised seizure		

Adapted with permission from the Commission of Classification and Terminology of the ILAE (1981)[214]

Table 1.2 (continued)

I. Generalised onset

A. Seizures with tonic and/or clonic manifestations
1. Tonic–clonic seizures
2. Clonic seizures
3. Tonic seizures

B. Absences
1. Typical absences
2. Atypical absences
3. Myoclonic absences

C. Myoclonic seizure types
1. Myoclonic seizures
2. Myoclonic–astatic seizures
3. Eyelid myoclonia

D. Epileptic spasms

E. Atonic seizures

II. Focal onset (partial)

A. Local
1. Neocortical
   (a) Without local spread
      (i) Focal clonic seizures
      (ii) Focal myoclonic seizures
      (iii) Inhibitory motor seizures
      (iv) Focal sensory seizures with elementary symptoms
      (v) Aphasic seizures
   (b) With local spread
      (i) Jacksonian march seizures
      (ii) Focal (asymmetrical) tonic seizures
      (iii) Focal sensory seizures with experiential symptoms
2. Hippocampal and parahippocampal

B. With ipsilateral propagation to:
1. Neocortical areas (includes hemiclonic seizures)
2. Limbic areas (includes gelastic seizures)

C. With contralateral spread to:
1. Neocortical areas (hyperkinetic seizures)
2. Limbic areas (dyscognitive seizures with or without automatisms [psychomotor])

D. Secondarily generalised
1. Tonic–clonic seizures
2. Absence seizures
3. Epileptic spasms (unverified)

III. Neonatal seizures

Reproduced with permission from Engel (2006)[215]
Table 1.3 Epileptic seizures

Syncopal Attacks Imitating Epileptic Seizures

2

Syncopes are among the most common non-epileptic attacks misdiagnosed as epileptic seizures, including GTCSs.[1,25-39]

A syncope is defined as a paroxysmal event of loss of consciousness and postural tone caused by cerebral hypoperfusion with spontaneous recovery.[38] There is an abrupt cutting off of the energy substrates to the cerebral cortex, usually through a sudden decrease in cerebral perfusion by oxygenated blood.[31] If cerebral perfusion/oxygenation is cut off for a period of 8–10 s, then a clinical picture comprising loss of consciousness and postural tone, pallor and sweating, brief (lasting seconds) extensor stiffening or spasms, and a few irregular myoclonic jerks of the limbs may occur. The whole episode is brief, usually lasting less than 10 s. There is a great variety in the amplitude of the myoclonic jerks, the degree of stiffening and the recovery time after syncope.[31]

Cerebral syncope is defined as a syncope that results from derangement of cerebral autoregulation leading to cerebral vasoconstriction with resultant cerebral hypoxia in the absence of systemic hypotension.

Convulsive syncope is a term used for any type of syncope manifesting with convulsive movements.

Prodromal warning symptoms (*presyncope*) are commonly present but sometimes these are only recalled when syncope is reproduced, as in the head-up tilt test. They develop over 1–5 min and include light headedness, nausea, a feeling of warmth, sweating, palpitation, greying or blacking of vision, muffled hearing and feeling distant. At this stage a syncope may be averted by lying down in a horizontal position with the head down and legs up. Lack of prodromal symptoms, such as in a tussive syncope, are explained by the rapidly developing cerebral hypoperfusion.

The setting and stimulus are the most important identifiable factors/precipitants in allowing the presumptive diagnosis of syncope. Simple faints or vasovagal syncope most often occur upon getting up quickly or after prolonged standing, particularly if associated with peripheral vasodilatation (e.g. hot, unventilated, crowded places, or after drug or alcohol use) or increased vagal tone (e.g. bloody, terrifying, or obnoxious scenes, and painful stimuli).

Cerebral hypoperfusion most commonly results from conditions that decrease venous return (e.g. reflex-mediated vasomotor instability) or disorders that decrease cardiac output, such as primary cardiac disorders.

C.P. Panayiotopoulos, *Imitators of Epileptic Seizures*,
DOI 10.1007/978-1-4471-4023-8_2, © Springer-Verlag London 2012

Precipitating factors or triggers such as upright position, bathroom, crowded and humid places, lack of food, unpleasant circumstances, venipuncture

Prodromal symptoms of cerebral ischaemia, such as dizziness, greying of vision and tinnitus

Gradual onset over seconds to 1 min

Pallor and sweating

Lack or rare occurrence of convulsions (other than myoclonic jerks), urinary incontinence or tongue biting

Brief duration (1–30 s)

Rapid recovery with no post-ictal confusion

Table 2.1 Commonly emphasised clinical manifestations of syncope

Convulsions occur in 70–90% of syncopes; symptoms include myoclonus, tonic flexion or extension, more complex movements and automatisms such as lip licking, chewing or fumbling

Visual hallucinations (a perception of grey haze, coloured patches, glaring lights or more complex scenes involving landscapes, familiar situations or people) and, less often, auditory hallucinations (rushing and roaring sounds, traffic and machine noises, and talking and screaming human voices, but never intelligible speech) are frequent (60%) in both convulsive and non-convulsive syncope[40]

Syncope usually happens in an upright position but may also occur in the supine position (e.g. venipuncture)

Sudden onset, urinary incontinence and trauma are not uncommon

Abdominal pain that may be confused with epigastric aura may occur at onset. Auras comprising epigastric, vertiginous, visual or somatosensory experiences occur both in neurally mediated and cardiogenic syncope[41]

Pallor and sweating are not invariable symptoms at onset and may be symptoms of autonomic epileptic seizures with or without secondarily GTCSs

Complete recovery may not be rapid and post-ictal confusion may occur, although neither of them reaches even close to the severity of that after a GTCS

Eyes, as in GTCSs, are always open during syncope and the most consistent oculomotor sign is an upward turning of the eyes early in its course, which may be followed by lateral eye deviation[42,43]

Table 2.2 Clinical features of syncopes not emphasised in their differentiation from epileptic seizures

In general, syncopes are categorised into:

- Neurally mediated syncopes (neurocardiogenic or reflex-mediated syncope) that are usually benign
- Cardiogenic syncopes from either cardiac rhythm or structural cardiac disorders, which are potentially life threatening

Autonomic disturbances may also lead to cerebral hypoperfusion and fainting as with orthostatic syncope.

In differentiating syncopes from GTCSs, textbooks usually emphasise the characteristics of typical syncopes that are listed in Table 2.1.

Based on a proper synthesis of the quality and chronological order of the clustering of these symptoms, the differential diagnosis of syncopes from GTCSs is rarely a problem. However, there are important points to consider and these are listed in Table 2.2.

Neurally Mediated Syncope

Examples of neurally mediated or non-cardiogenic syncopes include:

- Vasovagal syncope (simple faint) – variants of which may include reflex anoxic seizures (reflex asystolic syncope) and cyanotic breath-holding attacks (of prolonged expiratory apnoea) in infants and children
- Situation-related syncope caused by increased intrathoracic pressure, as a result of, for example, cough (tussive syncope), Valsalva manoeuvres, or straining to void (micturition syncope) or defecate
- Carotid sinus syncope

Vasovagal Syncope

Vasovagal syncope is the most common and familiar form of neurally mediated syncope and results from a combination of excessive vagal tone, abnormal catecholamine response to stress, venous pooling during an upright stance and impaired cardiac filling. Episodes may begin in infancy, sometimes with reflex anoxic seizures, and thereafter are seen at all ages, although it predominates in otherwise normal children and adolescents. The frequency of vasovagal syncopes varies considerably from one to two during a lifetime to as common as more than once a day.

Reflex Anoxic Seizures

Reflex anoxic seizures (synonyms: pallid breath-holding attacks, pallid infantile syncope) are reflex asystolic syncopes in young children. An unexpected bump to the head, an occasional fright or seeing blood triggers a neurally mediated vagal discharge leading to severe bradycardia, asystole, syncope and anoxic seizure. The child falls unconscious, white as a sheet and looks dead.

Useful Clinical Note

Breath-holding attacks in children

In children, there are two main types of so-called 'breath-holding attacks':

- Cyanotic or blue breath-holding attacks (prolonged expiratory apnoea usually without syncope)
- Pallid or white breath-holding attacks (reflex anoxic seizures, which are reflex asystolic syncopes)

The term 'breath-holding' has been discouraged by Stephenson and Zuberi because it erroneously implies a voluntary action to obtain gains or a behavioural disorder; psychological disorders in those afflicted do not differ from those in control children.[37] In contrast to voluntary breath holding that occurs during inspiration, cyanotic breath-holding attacks occur during expiration.

The cyanotic or blue breath-holding attacks, which are more common than the pallid forms, are purely respiratory consisting of prolonged expiratory apnoea without any change in cardiac rate or rhythm. Attacks of prolonged expiratory apnoea have similar triggers to reflex anoxic seizures, but they usually occur when the child has reasons to suddenly become angry or frustrated or fearful. The child stops breathing and becomes cyanotic until spontaneous recovery with a deep breath.

Mixed breath-holding of expiratory apnoea and a degree of bradycardia or cardiac asystole occur.[37]

Clarification on Terminology

- Reflex anoxic seizures are syncopes (and not epileptic seizures).
- Anoxic epileptic seizures are epileptic seizures caused by syncopes.
- Cyanotic or blue breath-holding attacks are not syncopes.

Orthostatic Syncope

Orthostatic syncope (autonomic failure) results from failure of normal mechanisms to compensate for the temporary decrease in venous return after standing.

Syncope occurs within seconds or minutes of becoming upright, especially when rising and after meals. Unlike with reflex vasovagal syncope, the skin stays warm, the pulse rate is unchanged despite the fall in blood pressure, and sweating is absent. Assuming a horizontal position results in complete recovery. Causes include autonomic dysfunction, cardiovascular disorders and drugs. Orthostatic syncope secondary to autonomic failure is rare in childhood. Dopamine β-decarboxylase deficiency is a possibility in such a clinical situation.

Syncopes Induced by Valsalva Manoeuvre

During a Valsalva manoeuvre (powerful effort to exhale against a closed glottis) increased intrathoracic pressure limits the venous return to the heart and increases vagal tone, resulting in decreased cardiac outflow and syncope.

Rarely, patients may have self-induced syncope by Valsalva manoeuvre. This particularly occurs in children with learning disabilities and Rett syndrome. The anoxic attacks may be severe.

Micturition Syncope

Micturition syncope is a reflex-mediated situational syncope usually occurring in men while standing for nighttime micturition.

Several mechanisms act in concert:
- Postural – standing on leaving a warm bed causing hypotension
- Straining – Valsalva manoeuvre increasing an already high nocturnal vagal tone, causing bradycardia
- Emptying bladder – abrupt decrease in stimulus to bladder stretch receptors causing reflex vasodilatation and hypotension

Carotid Sinus Syncope

Carotid sinus hypersensitivity is a common cause of unexplained falls in elderly people of over 50 years of age.[44,45] The incidence steeply increases with age. Activation of one or both carotid sinuses causes peripheral vasodilation, hypotension and syncope in people with carotid sinus hypersensitivity. Clinical attacks of syncope or falls without definite loss of consciousness are attributed to carotid sinus pressure by head turning or tight collars. Some patients may suffer from orthostatic hypotension but usually there is no evidence of sympathetic or parasympathetic failure.

> *Diagnostic carotid sinus massage may be positive in asymptomatic elderly patients[45] and carries a risk of prolonged asystole, transient or permanent neurological deficit, stroke and sudden death.*

Cardiogenic Syncopes

Cardiogenic syncopes result from either rhythm (e.g. tachyarrhythmias or bradyarrhythmias) or structural (e.g. aortic or mitral stenosis, intracardiac tumours, cardiomyopathy, ischaemic heart disease) cardiac disorders. Cardiogenic syncopes are potentially life threatening and may be treatable. Morbidity and mortality is up to 50% within the first 3 years following the initial attack, and it is cause-dependent.

Palpitations, chest pain, shortness of breath, extreme fatigue or other features of cardiovascular insufficiency occur with other presyncopal symptoms of simple faints. Cardiac syncopes occur from any posture (e.g. arrhythmogenic syncope is common in bed), and during periods of high exertion or emotion. Anoxic seizures precipitated by exercise require the urgent exclusion of cardiac causes, although most turn out to be neurally mediated syncopes.

In tachyarrhythmias, a heart rate of more than 150–180 beats/min prevents adequate ventricular filling. In bradyarrhythmias, a heart rate of less than 30–35 beats/min prevents adequate cardiac output.

Attacks due to transient complete heart block are abrupt and short with rapid loss of consciousness. Lack of cardiac output may be due to short episodes of ventricular tachycardia or fibrillation. Prolongation of the QT interval may lead to such events. Attacks may be preceded by palpitations, extreme fatigue or presyncopal features. Mitral valve prolapse and aortic stenosis may present with episodic loss of awareness due to fluctuating cardiac output or associated arrhythmias. Aortic stenosis and hypertrophic cardiomyopathy is especially prone to episodes of sudden collapse with loss of awareness during exercise. Sometimes ventricular tachyarrhythmias occur with normal QT intervals.

The Long QT Syndrome

Of various cardiogenic syncopes, the long QT syndrome is of particular significance because it may be associated with convulsive syncopes that cause unexplained sudden death in a young person and closely imitate GTCSs. It is often of autosomal dominant inheritance with mutations in genes encoding potassium or sodium channels, depending on lineage. The mechanism of the syncope is a ventricular tachyarrhythmia, normally torsades de pointes triggered by fear or fright, particularly during exercise (especially when that exercise is emotionally charged) and during sleep.

The ECG is diagnostic. Genetic testing is available.

> *A 33-year-old apparently normal man had, over a period of 6 months, three unwitnessed rather severe falls due to loss of consciousness that resulted in head trauma. All of them occurred while cycling or jogging in days that he recalls were particularly intense. EEG was normal but a synchronous ECG showed long QT syndrome, verified with appropriate cardiological evaluation.*

Brugada syndrome, characterised by 3 types of ST-segment abnormalities, is another genetic ion channelopathy (usually SCN5A mutation) that may imitate epileptic attacks and other causes of sudden death. Genetic testing is available.

Useful Note

A proper ECG should be obtained in any patients suspected or newly diagnosed with epilepsy. Misdiagnosis of cardiac diseases as epilepsy is common and often difficult to recognise on clinical information alone. Therefore a proper ECG is mandatory for this crucial differentiation. Also consider that the adverse cardiac effects of some AEDs may have fatal consequences for patients with conditions such as long QT or Brugada syndrome and other disorders of cardiac conductivity.

Syncopes Induced by Drugs and Electrolyte Abnormalities

Drugs and electrolyte abnormalities are common causes of syncope secondarily to cardiac rhythm changes or autonomic disturbances. Some examples include beta-blockers, quinidine, calcium channel blockers, digoxin, hypomagnesaemia and hypokalaemia.

Syncopal Attacks Provoking Epileptic Seizures: Anoxic Epileptic Seizures

Occasionally, but likely more often than is reported, true epileptic seizures are triggered by non-epileptic syncopes in children and adults.[39,46] This combination of syncope and epileptic seizure has been called an *anoxic epileptic seizure* (do not confuse with reflex anoxic seizure, which is a syncope). Of anoxic epileptic seizures documented with home video recordings, examples include a neurally mediated syncope inducing a long, clonic epileptic seizure with some features of myoclonic absence, and a compulsive Valsalva manoeuvre in an older autistic child provoking a vibratory tonic epileptic seizure.[46]

Epileptic Seizures Imitating Syncope

Epileptic seizures may manifest with syncopal-like attacks which are common in Panayiotopoulos syndrome.[46a]

Psychogenic NEPEs Imitating Epileptic Seizures

3

Psychogenic NEPEs (PNEPEs) or psychogenic non-epileptic seizures are among the most common recurrent paroxysmal seizure-imitating events that result from a variety of psychological disturbances.[2,6,47-49] Their synonym 'pseudoseizures' is discouraged because it is considered prejudicial. PNEPEs are not 'pseudo' in that they are extremely real episodes and 'pseudo' implies a disparaging element for the event. Similar to epileptic seizures, PNEPEs can be very troublesome to a person's life and have their own stigma.

Patients with PNEPEs often experience severe depression, anxiety, emotional stress, rage, fear and panic, in addition to other mental disturbances. Conversion disorder is the most common cause of PNEPEs.[50] Other causes, with natural histories and treatments different from those of conversion disorder, include anxiety, dissociative, depersonalisation, somatisation, panic and psychotic disorders.[2,6,47-49] Factitious PNEPEs, including Munchausen syndrome, are sometimes difficult to diagnose and prove.

According to the fourth edition of the *Diagnostic and Statistical Manual of Mental Disorders* (DSM-IV)[51] psychological causes of physical symptoms are categorised as:

- Somatoform disorders
- Factitious disorders
- Malingering

Somatoform disorders are the unconscious production of physical symptoms due to psychological factors, which means that the symptoms are not under voluntary control. Patients with somatoform disorders are not faking illness; they sincerely believe that they have a serious physical problem. Specific somatoform disorders include:

- Somatisation disorder
- Conversion disorder
- Pain disorder
- Hypochondriasis
- Body dysmorphic disorder

Somatisation disorder is a relatively rare disorder that is associated with high medical resource utilisation.

In factitious disorders and malingering there is a conscious production of physical symptoms, in which individuals present with an illness that is deliberately produced or falsified. However, in factitious disorders patients intentionally act physically or mentally ill due to psychological factors of pathological needs without obvious benefits. Conversely, in malingering, patients fake an illness for a clear motive and benefit such as financial gain.

C.P. Panayiotopoulos, *Imitators of Epileptic Seizures*, DOI 10.1007/978-1-4471-4023-8_3, © Springer-Verlag London 2012

Often precipitated by stressful circumstances (stress is also a precipitating factor in epilepsies)

Can be induced in response to suggestion (useful in diagnostic provocative activating techniques; also called 'inductions')[55]

Occur in wakefulness and in the presence of witnesses (not unusual in epilepsies)

Lack stereotypical characteristics

'Convulsions' consist of asynchronous, asymmetrical, waxing and waning, accelerating and decelerating, convulsive-like movements, often with pelvic thrusts, flailing and tremors. These may be interrupted or resistant to restraint, and imitate seizures from the supplementary somatosensory area and are not GTCSs

Eyes are commonly closed (probably the most important symptom to enable differentiation from GTCSs and syncopes, where the eyes are invariably open)

Attempts to open the eyes passively often result in tightening of the eyelids (this may also occur infrequently in post-ictal confusion after a GTCS)

'Give-way weakness' on examination is common[55]

Consciousness may be retained throughout or shows marked fluctuations

There is no actual post-ictal confusion. The patient may become emotional and cry after the end of the non-epileptic seizure (this symptom is not unusual in patients with epileptic seizures)

Post-ictal behaviour of responding to questions in a whispered voice or responding to commands with partial motor responses is common and may be helpful in the diagnosis of PNEPEs[56]

Intractable to anti-epileptic medication (also occurring in epilepsies)

Belle indifference: Paradoxical lack of concern about the seizures, which contrasts to the emotional distress and behaviours exhibited during the attacks

Table 3.1 Diagnostic clues for convulsive psychogenic non-epileptic events (the more common of the PNEPEs)

Somatoform PNEPEs are much more common than malingering and factitious disorders.

PNEPEs, including staring spells,[52,53] are often extremely difficult to differentiate from epileptic seizures[2,6,47-49,54] and, conversely, certain types of epileptic seizures, such as those of mesial frontal lobe origin, masquerade as psychogenic-like attacks.

Table 3.1 provides some key diagnostic clues for recognising convulsive PNEPEs.

Convulsive Psychogenic Status Epilepticus

Convulsive psychogenic status epilepticus (commonly referred to as convulsive pseudostatus epilepticus) is common in patients with PNEPEs and it is often misdiagnosed as genuine and life-threatening convulsive status epilepticus.[57-60] These patients frequently have multiple episodes of 'status' and receive intensive care unit management. They usually have a history of other unexplained illness and deliberate self-poisoning. Episodes of anticonvulsant-induced respiratory arrest may occur.[57-60]

Diagnostic Traps

At least one of the usual signs associated with a GTCS (tongue biting, falling or incontinence) is reported by about a third of the patients with non-epileptic seizures.[61]

An ictal EEG is not always abnormal during epileptic seizures.

Psychogenic non-epileptic syncope (*synonyms: psychogenic pseudosyncope, hysterical fainting*) is a term used to include NEPEs with clinical manifestations of psychogenic origin that mimic syncope.[62] Patients suffer frequently recurrent syncopal-like episodes of 'limp, motionless fainting' with eyes closed, unresponsiveness and a normal EEG, including normal alpha rhythm. This is often associated with complaints of vertigo and with greater reported disability. The condition may be underdiagnosed and often remains misdiagnosed for many years. Patients may go through lengthy and sometimes invasive diagnostic procedures. The psychogenic non-epileptic syncope can be easily elicited by induction.[62]

Useful Clinical Notes

Look at the eyes and make the diagnosis

When eyes are closed during a paroxysmal event of convulsions with loss of consciousness, the probability (almost a certainty) is that this is a PNEPE. Eyes remain open or become open, if not previously open, during GTCSs and syncopes.

Try to passively open the eyes and make the diagnosis

The eyes may be closed in post-ictal states of epileptic seizures or other causes of organic impairment of consciousness. In these cases the eyes can usually be passively opened without resistance as opposed to PNEPEs where attempts to passively open the eyes are met with resistance or tightening of the eyelids.

Suffocation in Munchausen Syndrome by Proxy[37,63-66]

Intentional suffocation of an infant is an uncommon but severe event. In this situation, an adult, usually the mother, suffering from Munchausen syndrome by proxy repeatedly suffocates the infant by either pressing a hand or some other material over the infant's mouth or presses the infant's face against the adult's chest, with a resultant syncope and anoxic seizure. The evolution is much longer than the usual anoxic seizures, but a definitive diagnosis requires unequivocal *covert* video-recording evidence.

Panic Attacks[67-69]

Panic attacks are of abrupt onset, manifesting with an intense sense of extreme fear often with concomitant symptoms of trembling, shortness of breath, heart palpitations, chest pain, sweating, dizziness, hyperventilation, paraesthesias, nausea or vomiting, or sensations of choking. Panic attacks are actually a fight-or-flight response occurring out of context or as a response to minimal provocative factors. Patients suffer from panic, other anxiety disorders or phobias. Psychogenic non-epileptic panic attacks should mainly be differentiated from simple focal seizures of mesial temporal lobe epilepsy (see Fig. 3.1).

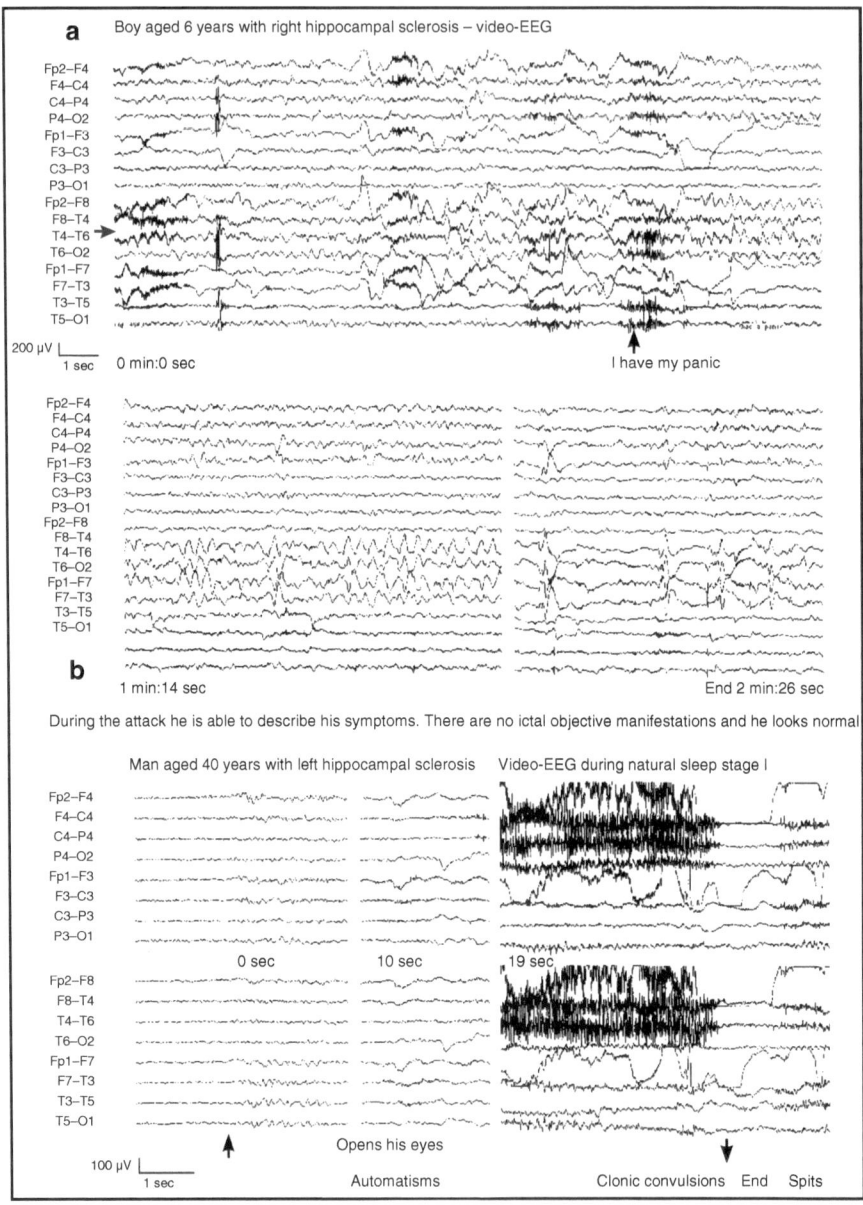

a Boy aged 6 years with right hippocampal sclerosis – video-EEG

200 µV | 1 sec   0 min:0 sec   I have my panic

b 1 min:14 sec   End 2 min:26 sec

During the attack he is able to describe his symptoms. There are no ictal objective manifestations and he looks normal

Man aged 40 years with left hippocampal sclerosis   Video-EEG during natural sleep stage I

0 sec   10 sec   19 sec

100 µV | 1 sec   Opens his eyes

Automatisms   Clonic convulsions   End   Spits

Fig. 3.1 (**a**) This was the second EEG of a boy aged 6 years, referred for episodes of panic attacks and a recent GTCS. The resting EEG was entirely normal but one of his seizures was recorded from onset (0 min:0 s; *red arrow*) and lasted for 2 min and 26 s. The child looked disturbed, complaining, 'I have my panic' (black arrow). He was able to communicate well during the whole seizure. Speech and cognition were normal. Brain MRI documented right hippocampal sclerosis. (**b**) Sample of video-EEG during a brief seizure of a man aged 40 years with increasing numbers of complex focal seizures typical of hippocampal epilepsy. The MRI documented left hippocampal sclerosis. Note that towards the end of the attack the patient had mild right-sided clonic convulsions (see muscle artefacts), although he never had a GTCS. Also note that he immediately spits after the cessation of the seizure

Hyperventilation Syndrome[70-73]

Hyperventilation syndrome is defined as:

A syndrome, characterized by a variety of somatic symptoms induced by physiologically inappropriate hyperventilation and usually reproduced by voluntary hyperventilation.[70]

Hyperventilation is defined as breathing in excess of the metabolic needs of the body, eliminating more carbon dioxide than is produced and, consequently, resulting in respiratory alkalosis and an elevated blood pH.

Hyperventilation may have organic or physiological causes, but the syndrome of hyperventilation is usually associated with emotional triggers and thoracic breathing tendency.

Hyperventilation syndrome is a frequent disorder probably affecting 6 % of the population, mainly aged 15–55 years old. Women are seven times more frequently affected than men. It occurs in acute (1 % of cases) and chronic forms.

The acute forms of hyperventilation syndrome manifest with agitation, hyperpnoea, tachypnoea and dyspnoea, chest pain, dizziness, palpitations, carpopedal spasm, paraesthesia, generalised weakness, a sense of suffocation and syncope. An emotionally stressful precipitating event can often be identified. Symptoms may be unilateral. The chest pain is often relieved rather than provoked by exercise. ECG abnormalities may occur and include prolonged QT interval, ST depression or elevation, and T-wave inversion.

The chronic hyperventilation syndrome presents with a galaxy of multi-system symptoms without any clinically apparent hyperventilatory respiratory pattern. Hypocapnoea and respiratory alkalosis develop rapidly upon the onset of hyperventilation and can be maintained by nearly imperceptible hyperventilation, such as by taking an occasional deep breath or frequent sighs interspersed with normal respirations, usually with thoracic muscle use.

The therapeutic approach includes psychological counselling, breathing exercises, physiotherapy and relaxation. Techniques of rebreathing into a paper bag are discouraged by some experts because significant hypoxia and death have been reported in patients with organic causes of hyperventilation. Simple reassurance and an explanation of how hyperventilation produces the symptoms is usually sufficient to terminate the episode. Physically compressing the upper thorax and having the patient exhale maximally decreases hyperinflation of the lungs. Instructing the patient to breathe abdominally, using the diaphragm more than the chest wall, often leads to improvement in subjective dyspnoea and eventually corrects many of the associated symptoms.

Management of PNEPEs

PNEPEs need urgent and skilful treatment, which is often successful, particularly if they are recognised and managed during the early stages.[2,6,49,74,75] The role of the physician is not just simply to announce to the patient: 'You do not suffer from epileptic seizures'. At this stage, the patient requires a thorough and tactful explanation of what this new diagnosis of PNEPE means and the appropriate management procedures. These patients have been allowed to believe for many years that they suffered from 'epilepsy' that was intractable to medication. Their reaction and that of their family to a new diagnosis of 'psychogenic seizures' (also taking into consideration the negative social implications and attitudes to this term) should be thoroughly considered. Patients' understanding and reactions to a diagnosis of these non-epileptic attacks are important factors that should contribute to the development of more tailored treatment approaches.[76]

> *Sensitivity to the patient, the use of a multidisciplinary team and the recognition that PNEPEs are as devastating as medically refractory epilepsy are critical to a successful treatment outcome.*[6]

Non-epileptic Paroxysmal Movement Disorders Imitating Epileptic Seizures

Non-epileptic paroxysmal movement disorders of whatever cause are common imitators of epileptic seizures and *vice versa*.

'WE MOVE' (Worldwide Education and Awareness for Movement Disorders; www.wemove.org/) is a highly recommended website source for excellent reviews, glossaries, and slide and video presentations for medical educational purposes. It also hosts the MDVU site (Movement Disorders Virtual University; www.mdvu.org).

Paroxysmal movement disorders are neurological disorders characterised by abrupt, transient episodes of abnormal involuntary movement, such as chorea, athetosis, dystonia and/or ballismus (paroxysmal dyskinesias) or impaired coordination of voluntary actions and other associated findings (paroxysmal ataxias). Depending upon the specific disorder, episodes may be precipitated or worsened by different factors. For example:

- In those with paroxysmal kinesigenic dyskinesia, episodes may be triggered by sudden voluntary movements
- In non-kinesigenic dyskinesia, episodes occur spontaneously and may be worsened by caffeine or alcohol consumption, stress, fatigue or other factors
- In patients with paroxysmal kinesigenic ataxias, episodes may be triggered by sudden voluntary movements or postural changes.

These disorders may be familial, appear to occur randomly for unknown reasons, or occur secondary to other underlying conditions or disorders.

Tics, Compulsions, Stereotypies and Mannerisms

Tics are intermittent, repeated, stereotyped movements or sounds that may occur in an infrequent or almost continuous manner. Tics may be 'simple', such as a cough, grunt, facial twitch or shoulder shrug, or 'complex', such as a word, phrase or a stereotyped sequence of movements. Tics are often made worse by stress, upset or demand for mental concentration. Tics last more than 200 ms with a frequency that may be altered voluntarily.

Tics are not voluntary movements, although they may be incorporated into an apparently voluntary gesture to avoid embarrassment.

Tic disorders frequently occur in association with compulsions and attention-deficit disorder.

C.P. Panayiotopoulos, *Imitators of Epileptic Seizures*,
DOI 10.1007/978-1-4471-4023-8_4, © Springer-Verlag London 2012

Compulsions are complex behaviours that respond to a psychological need, such as hand washing due to a fear of germs. The actions 'feel' voluntary, but the patient may describe a sense of fear or impending doom if the action is not performed. Compulsions are frequently associated with obsessions, tics or Tourette's syndrome.

Stereotypies are repetitive, stereotyped, purposeless movements that may be made by normal children when they are bored, excited or engrossed in an activity. Stereotypies are often associated with attention-deficit disorder, developmental delay or autism. They may consist of hand flapping, clapping, slapping, fluttering, rocking or facial movements. These children are not necessarily aware that they are making the movements. In some cases, these movements can be voluntarily suppressed.

Mannerisms are normal voluntary phenomena; i.e. the particular movement accompaniments that people develop while performing certain movements or gestures. They may appear abnormal, particularly if the mannerism involves unusual or unnecessary postures. The subjects can modify them by command.

Tremor

In tremor the contraction is bidirectional, affects agonist and antagonist muscles alternatively, and is more rhythmic than myoclonus; however, the phenomenological border between tremor and myoclonus is sometimes unclear (e.g. recently some authorities have categorised palatal myoclonus as tremor rather than myoclonus,[77] and further, in some neurodegenerative disorders, the initial stages of action in myoclonus may in fact be small amplitude tremor).[77]

Non-epileptic Movement Disorders in Neonates and Infants Imitating Seizures

Non-epileptic movement disorders in neonates and infants may be misdiagnosed as epileptic seizures. The description of the following conditions are based on a recent review by Vigevano[78] with video presentations of these events.

Jitteriness[78]
Jitteriness manifests with involuntary rhythmic movements of rapid alternating contraction of agonist and antagonist muscles at 4 or 5 Hz with equal intensity. It may be symmetrical or asymmetrical, involves mainly limbs and commonly occurs in the first days or months of age. Jitteriness may be spontaneous, or is stimulus-triggered and mainly occurs when the child cries. It can be terminated by passive flexion of the affected limb. Jitteriness tends to remit within the fourth and fifth months of life.

Jitteriness occurs in normal children but is more frequent in those with perinatal ischaemic encephalopathy or preterm babies with dyselectrolytaemia or hypoglycaemia. Children whose mothers have taken sedatives during pregnancy are vulnerable. Hypertonia, hyperexcitability and persistence of primitive reflexes can be observed.

Tonic Reflex Seizures of Early Infancy[79]

This is an episodic benign movement disorder of healthy, mainly male babies aged between 2 and 3 months. Attacks manifest with tonic contraction with extension of four limbs, apnoea and cyanosis, without loss of consciousness. They last for 3–10 s. They are triggered by movement or tactile stimulation and occur only when the child is awake and held in a vertical position by an adult. Ictal and inter-ictal EEG are normal. Spontaneous remission occurs within 2 months of onset.

Alternating Hemiplegia[78]

This is a very rare and severe disease of unknown aetiology. It starts in the first few months of age. Episodes of hemiplegia have a duration ranging from a few minutes to several hours. They are often preceded by other paroxysmal manifestations, such as short periods of muscle hypertonia or monocular nystagmus. Hemiplegia alternates from one to the other side but may also affect both sides simultaneously. The attack begins with a deviation of the head towards the hemiplegic side of the body and progresses to hemiplegia, causing difficulty with swallowing and breathing. Attacks last for hours or sometimes several days, and recur with a frequency of more than one attack per month. The baby shows full recovery after sleep. Children develop severe motor and mental deficits. Epileptic seizures may appear in late infancy. Brain imaging is normal. EEG shows unilateral slow waves. Anti-migraine and AEDs prove to be ineffective.

Benign Paroxysmal Torticollis[78]

This consists of lateral head deviation sometimes associated with trunk torsion and paroxysmal crying. It may alternate from side to side. It ranges from several seconds to hours in duration. Attacks are often accompanied by vomiting, pallor, and ataxia, settling spontaneously within hours or days. Onset is generally in early infancy, and attacks may be frequent but remit before the age of 2 years. Some patients may later develop paroxysmal vertigo, migraine and transient episodic ataxia.

Rhythmic Behavioural Movements[78]

Normal children, especially when feeling pleasure and joy, may manifest rhythmic movements of the head and neck. These start, with a variable frequency, around the age of 1 year and remit by the age of 2 or 3 years.

Self-gratification Disorder[80]

Gratification disorder, otherwise called infantile masturbation, is an important consideration in the differential diagnosis of epilepsy and other paroxysmal events in early childhood. Median age at onset is 10 months (range: 3 months to 5 years) with several episodes per week. There may be direct genital stimulation but other manoeuvres, particularly involving flexion and adduction of the thighs, may achieve the same effect. Types of behaviour manifested include dystonic posturing, grunting, rocking, eidetic imagery and sweating. Cyanosis, lip smacking, staring, shaking, pallor, giggling and appearing frightened/in discomfort are also reported. Infantile masturbation takes place in a variety of situations and is particularly common in car seats. The children can usually be distracted during the episodes, often appearing annoyed, and may quickly resume the activity. The diagnosis can usually be secured by taking a detailed history. Video recordings, usually easily obtained, are very helpful.

Gastro-oesophageal Reflux in Infants

Gastro-oesophageal reflux disease is the passage of gastric contents into the oesophagus. This is a normal physiological process including regurgitation (passage of gastric contents up to the mouth). It peaks between 1 and 4 months of age, and usually resolves by 6–12 months of age.

Gastro-oesophageal reflux disease is a pathological process in infants manifested by poor weight gain, signs of oesophagitis, persistent respiratory symptoms and neurobehavioural changes. These are unlikely to imitate epileptic seizures. However, in infants some gastro-oesophageal reflux attacks may sometimes impose diagnostic problems.[39] Babies cannot complain of heartburn, but they may cry and have disturbed sleep. There may be significant vomiting with poor weight gain and risk of aspiration. Approximately 85% of infants vomit during the first week of life and another 10% have symptoms by 6 weeks of age. Symptoms abate without treatment in 60% of infants by 2 years of age, as these infants begin to assume an upright position and eat solid foods. Reflux may cause wheeze and cough. In premature babies it can cause apnoea and bradycardia.

Sandifer syndrome manifests with brief (about 1–3 min) NEPEs of dystonic posturing associated with gastro-oesophageal reflux; hiatal hernia is common. The attacks consist of sudden torticollis, with arching of the back and rigid opisthotonic posturing, mainly involving the neck, back and upper extremities. During the attack, the infant may become very quiet or, less commonly, become very distressed and uncomfortable. Agitation is most commonly observed as the dystonic posturing abates. Sandifer syndrome occurs from infancy to early childhood with a peak at age 18–36 months. Children with severe mental impairment or spasticity may experience Sandifer syndrome in late childhood to adolescence. Sandifer syndrome is most commonly mistaken for seizures. However, NEPEs of Sandifer syndrome occur within 1 h of feeding, often following an imposed change of posture and the babies frequently have a history of vomiting, failure to thrive and repeated chest infections. The EEG is normal. A barium oesophagogram, oesophagoscopy or a pH probe may demonstrate the reflux.

Benign Neonatal Sleep Myoclonus

Benign neonatal sleep myoclonus is a common non-epileptic condition misdiagnosed as epileptic myoclonic seizures or sometimes as infantile spasms. The myoclonus occurs during non-rapid eye movement (NREM) sleep in otherwise normal neonates.[81-83] It mainly affects the distal parts of the upper extremities. The lower limbs and axial muscles are less often involved. The myoclonic jerks – synchronous or asynchronous, unilateral or bilateral, mild or violent – are fast and usually last for 10–20 s. Occasionally they may occur in repetitive clusters of 2 or 3 s for 30 min or longer imitating myoclonic status epilepticus or a series of epileptic fits. The myoclonic jerks may get worse by gentle restraint. They abruptly stop when the child is awakened. Sleep is not disturbed.

There are no other clinical manifestations like those accompanying neonatal seizures, such as apnoea, autonomic disturbances, automatisms, eye deviation, oral–buccal–lingual movements or crying.

Neurological mental state and development are normal.

Aetiology: This is unknown and the condition does not appear to be familial. The myoclonus is likely to be generated in the brain stem.

Diagnostic procedures: The diagnosis is based on clinical features. All relevant laboratory studies, including sleep EEG during the myoclonus, are normal.

Differential diagnosis: Benign neonatal sleep myoclonus should be easy to differentiate from relevant epileptic disorders in this age group by its occurrence in normal neonates and only during sleep. When in doubt, a normal sleep EEG during the myoclonus is confirmatory of this non-epileptic condition.

Prognosis: The prognosis is excellent with the myoclonus commonly remitting by the age of 2–7 months.

Management: There is no need for any treatment, although minute doses of clonazepam before bed are often beneficial. Other AEDs are contraindicated.

Benign Non-epileptic Myoclonus of Early Infancy (Fejerman Syndrome)

This syndrome, which has recently been thoroughly re-assessed,[16] is a paroxysmal non-epileptic movement disorder of otherwise healthy infants who have normal EEG and development. The name 'Fejerman syndrome' has been proposed[17] to replace various unsatisfactory descriptive terms such as 'benign non-epileptic infantile spasms' or 'shuddering attacks'.[18,84,85]

Demographic data: Peak age at onset is from 1–12 (peak at 6) months. Boys slightly predominate (59%).

Clinical manifestations: The attacks are sudden and brief (1–2 s) and consist of spasms or tonic contractions (38%), shuddering (35%), myoclonus

(23%), atonia or negative myoclonus, combined (9%). They affect the head and neck, upper limbs and trunk muscles. They are usually symmetrical and in flexion. Less frequently, there may be flexion, abduction or adduction of the elbows and knees and extension or elevation of the arms. They do not involve localised muscle groups and there are no focal or lateralising features. The attacks are often repeated at frequent and brief intervals several times a day but not necessarily every day; 40% occur in clusters. The intensity varies from mild attacks, which are most usual, to severe attacks mimicking infantile spasms, which occur less frequently. Attacks mainly occur while the babies are awake but in 15% of babies they occur both while awake and during sleep. Excitement, fear, anger, frustration or the need to move the bowels or to void are precipitating factors.

Aetiology: Fejerman syndrome is of unknown aetiology. Non-epileptic paroxysmal movements may result from an exaggeration of physiological myoclonus.[18]

Diagnostic procedures: The diagnosis is based on clinical features. All relevant laboratory studies including sleep- and awake-stage EEGs during the spasms are normal.

Differential diagnosis: The main differential diagnosis is from epileptic spasms that may share similar clinical features. A normal ictal and inter-ictal EEG in benign non-epileptic infantile spasms is of decisive significance.

Prognosis: Fejerman syndrome has a good prognosis, with spontaneous remission usually occurring by age 2 or 3 years. There is no increase in the incidence of epilepsy or developmental delay.

Management: There is no convincing evidence of any beneficial treatment. AEDs are unnecessary and potentially harmful.[18]

Hyperekplexia

Hyperekplexia (*synonym: familial startle disease*) is the first human disease shown to result from mutations within a neurotransmitter gene.[86,87]

Demographic data: Onset ranges from intra-uterine life or birth, to later at any time from the neonatal period to adulthood. Both sexes are equally affected. It is a rare disorder. Only approximately 150 cases have been reported.

Clinical manifestations: Clinically, hyperekplexia is characterised by:

- Pathological and excessive startle responses to unexpected auditory or tactile stimuli (e.g. sudden noise, movement or touch)
- Severe generalised stiffness (i.e. hypertonia in flexion, which disappears in sleep).

The startle response is characterised by a sudden generalised muscular rigidity and resistance to habituation. In babies, the muscle stiffening often causes respiratory impairment and apnoea that may be fatal. In older patients, the startle response causes frequent falls, like a log, without loss of consciousness.

If an unborn baby is affected the mother may first notice abnormal intra-uterine movements. In neonates, apnoea and sluggish feeding efforts occur as a consequence of episodic extreme stiffening during the first 24 h of life. After the first 24 h, surviving infants exhibit the hyperekplexic startle response to nose tapping, which is a useful diagnostic test.

Clinical phenotypic expression varies from mild to very severe forms.

The minor forms manifest with excessive but often mild startle responses, but without hypertonia. In infancy these are facilitated by febrile illness, whereas in adults these are facilitated by emotional stress.

In the major forms affected neonates have hypertonia and marked startle responses that result in falls. There is no impairment of consciousness, but the patient remains temporarily stiff after the attack.

Sleep episodic shaking of the limbs (nocturnal or sleep myoclonus) resembling generalised clonus or repetitive myoclonus is often prominent, lasting for minutes with no impairment of consciousness. The jerks are spontaneous arousal reactions.

Neurologically, there is generalised muscle hypertonia–stiffness, hence the term *stiff baby syndrome* (which is probably the same disease as hyperekplexia).[88] Gait may be unstable, insecure and puppet-like. Brain-stem and tendon reflexes are exaggerated.

Umbilical and inguinal hernias, presumably due to increased intra-abdominal pressure, are common.

Aetiology: Hyperekplexia is usually inherited as an autosomal dominant and less often recessive trait. It is due to mutations within the *GLRA1* gene on chromosome 5q31-33, which encodes the alpha 1 subunit of the glycine receptor.[89-91] The minor form of hyperekplexia is usually sporadic and seldom due to a genetic defect in the *GLRA1* gene.[87]

Diagnostic procedures: The nose tap test is the most useful test. Tapping the tip of the nose of an unaffected baby will elicit either a blink response or no response, but in hyperekplexia there is a distinct startle response, which is repeated each time the nose is tapped.

The EEG of startle responses in hyperekplexia is normal.[92] A slowing of background activity with eventual flattening may occur, but this corresponds to the phase of apnoea, bradycardia and cyanosis.[92]

Differential diagnosis: Hyperekplexia in the neonatal period may be misdiagnosed as one of the following disorders: congenital stiffman syndrome, startle epilepsy, myoclonic seizures, neonatal tetany, cerebral palsy or drug (phenothiazine) toxicity. Accurate recognition of hyperekplexia in a newborn is important in order to initiate early and appropriate treatment, which may be life saving.

Prognosis: This is generally good in treated patients. Untreated infants experience recurring apnoea until 1 year of age. The exaggerated startle response persists to adulthood. Hypertonia gradually improves during the course of the first and second year of life and tone is usually almost normal by the age of 3 years. Hypertonia may recur in adult life.

Management: There is a dramatic response to clonazepam (0.1–0.2 mg/kg/day).[93] A simple manoeuvre to terminate the startle response is forcibly flexing the baby by pressing the head towards the knees. This may be life saving when prolonged stiffness impedes respiration. Affected families are advised to seek genetic counselling.

Other Non-epileptic Paroxysmal Movement Disorders

Familial Paroxysmal Dystonic Choreoathetosis

Familial paroxysmal dystonic choreoathetosis (synonyms: paroxysmal non-kinesigenic dyskinesia, paroxysmal non-kinesigenic dystonia [Mount-Reback syndrome]) is a non-epileptic hyperkinetic movement disorder linked to chromosome 2q35. It is characterised by attacks of involuntary chorea, dystonia and ballism with onset in childhood.[94-96] Attacks typically last from half an hour to several hours (with no signs of abnormality between attacks) and may occur several times each week. There is no impairment of consciousness and the EEG is normal during the episodes. Attacks are precipitated by a variety of factors, including caffeine, alcohol and emotion. Contrary to frontal lobe seizures, attacks in familial paroxysmal dystonic choreoathetosis can be relieved by short periods of sleep in most subjects.

Non-epileptic Paroxysmal Kinesigenic Choreoathetosis[97-100]

Non-epileptic paroxysmal kinesigenic choreoathetosis is characterised by recurrent, brief attacks of involuntary movements induced by sudden voluntary movements. The involuntary movements combine tonic, dystonic and choreoathetoid features on one or both sides. They are often associated with dysarthria, upwards gaze and sensory aura. Consciousness is entirely intact. Their duration is usually 10–30 s and no more than 3 min. The EEG during the attacks is normal. There may be tens of attacks per day in more than half of patients. Onset is in the mid-teens with a range of 5–16 years. Most patients respond well to AEDs, such as carbamazepine, phenytoin or phenobarbital.[101] In nearly all patients, spontaneous remissions occur between 20 and 30 years of age.

Paroxysmal kinesigenic choreoathetosis is distinct from reflex epilepsy. However, patients may have a history of benign infantile seizures between the ages of 3 and 8 months.[102,103] There are no differences in the clinical presentation of cases with and without infantile seizures.[102] In addition, there may be a family history of epileptic seizures in 8% of cases.

Non-epileptic paroxysmal choreoathetosis may also be induced by exercise.

A 9-year-old child was referred for a second EEG because of a 'history of left-sided focal motor seizures, which recently increased. Previous EEG showed non-specific paroxysmal abnormalities'. Intelligent history taking and application of 'seizure' provocation by the EEG technologist allowed a definite diagnosis of exercise-induced paroxysmal choreoathetosis. After establishing by history taking that the events were induced by exercise, the child was asked to exercise and this induced three typical attacks which were video-EEG recorded. These were brief (under 2 min) episodes of asymmetrical dystonia, choreoathetosis and ballistic movements.

Paroxysmal kinesigenic choreoathetosis, paroxysmal exercise-induced choreoathetosis/dystonia and benign infantile seizures map to the same region on chromosome 16, suggesting that they may be allelic disorders.

Episodic Ataxia Type 1

Of the various types of episodic ataxias,[104,105] only type 1 may cause problems for differential diagnosis. In episodic ataxia type 1, patients suffer from brief attacks of ataxia and dysarthria, lasting seconds to minutes, often associated with continuous inter-attack myokymia. Attacks are diurnal and may occur several times per day. The EEG is frequently abnormal and patients may also have seizures. Episodic ataxia type 1 is a rare, autosomal dominant, potassium channelopathy caused by different point mutations in the voltage-gated potassium channel gene *KCNA1* on chromosome 12p13.[106,107]

A 19-year-old intelligent woman was erroneously diagnosed as having epileptic seizures. She had brief, for less than 1 min, episodes of ataxia and dysarthria since approximately the age of 10 years. She has three types of attacks:

- The most common type is in her legs. She feels this coming and then her legs 'cannot obey her any more'.
- The second type is restricted in the upper extremities. Again, she feels this coming soon before marked cerebellar type of symptoms in the hands.
- The third type are clear cut attacks of dysarthria. She can initially be understood, but later within seconds her speech is incomprehensible.

In some occasions, there is a successive progression of the symptoms from the legs to the arms and to the speech. The latter episodes are longer, for up to a maximum of 5 min. On no occasion was there impairment of consciousness or inability to recognise her surroundings or to understand people talking to her. Over the years, these episodes appeared to become more frequent (two per week), more apparent and longer in duration. In addition, she started having episodes of marked positional tremor and attacks of periorbital and perioral myokymia.

Series of EEG were abnormal with bursts of sharp–slow-waves bilaterally in the mid-temporal regions. Brain MRI was normal. Molecular analysis revealed the first truncation to be reported in the KCNA1 gene (C1249T).[107]

Non-epileptic Severe Amnesic and Confusional Attacks Imitating Epileptic Seizures

5

Non-epileptic severe amnesic attacks and lengthy confusional episodes may be misdiagnosed as epileptic seizures or non-convulsive status epilepticus (focal or generalised).

Transient epileptic amnesia refers to transient global amnesia of ictal or post-ictal epileptic origin. This is usually briefer and more frequent than transient global amnesia and patients frequently have complaints of 'memory gaps' in their medical history; these 'gaps' are usually caused by complex focal seizures. Pure amnestic epileptic seizures sometimes occur in patients with temporal lobe epilepsy but they never represent the only type of seizure in these patients.[108]

Pure amnestic seizures are defined as seizures during which the only clinical manifestation is the patients' inability to retain in their memory what occurs during the seizure coupled with the preservation of other cognitive functions and the ability to interact normally with their physical and social environment. It is postulated that they result from selective and usually bilateral ictal inactivation of mesial temporal structures without isocortical involvement. In most instances pure amnestic seizures can be distinguished from episodes of transient global amnesia on clinical grounds.[108]

Transient Global Amnesia[109-111]

Transient global amnesia is a clinical syndrome characterised by a sudden, short-term profound deficit of anterograde and often retrograde memory without any other focal neurological signs or symptoms. Patients may repeatedly ask questions concerning transpiring events and appear agitated and confused. Personal identity, attention, visual-spatial skills and social skills are retained. Symptoms typically last less than 24 hours (median 4 hours). As the attack resolves, the amnesia improves, but the patient has complete or severe permanent amnesia of intra-attack events.

Transient global amnesia usually affects middle-aged or elderly men. In men, they occur more frequently after a physical precipitating event. In women, episodes are mainly associated with an emotional precipitating event, a history of anxiety and a pathological personality. In younger patients, a history of headaches may constitute an important risk factor. The cause is

C.P. Panayiotopoulos, *Imitators of Epileptic Seizures*,
DOI 10.1007/978-1-4471-4023-8_5, © Springer-Verlag London 2012

unclear; a history of migraine is common in younger patients. No link is found with vascular risk factors.

Transient global amnesia should be differentiated from epileptic seizures, drug intoxication and psychogenic fugue.

Transient global amnesia of any cause is attributed to transient dysfunction in limbic–hippocampal circuits (or in the basal forebrain cholinergic inputs to that circuitry). It can be considered a model for a focal transient perturbation of memory circuits in the temporomesial region.

Psychogenic (Dissociative) Fugues

Psychogenic (dissociative) fugues consist of an inability to recall some or all of one's past combined with either loss of identity or the formation of a new identity. They result from trauma or stress. They often manifest with sudden, unexpected, purposeful travel away from home. Diagnosis is based on medical history after ruling out other causes of amnesia. The incidence of dissociative fugue increases in connection with wars, accidents and natural disasters. Fugues are often mistaken for malingering, because fugues may remove the person from accountability for his actions, absolve him of certain responsibilities or reduce his exposure to hazardous situations. However, fugues are spontaneous, unplanned and not faked. Most fugues are brief and self-limited. Impairment after the fugue ends is usually mild and short-lived.

Prolonged Confusional States

Prolonged confusional states of acute encephalopathy have many causes such as diabetic ketoacidosis, hypoglycaemia, respiratory, renal or hepatic failure, hyperpyrexia, sepsis and drug poisoning. They may be the predominant features of encephalitis, meningitis, head injury and cerebrovascular accidents. Some disorders such as porphyria and urea cycle enzyme defects may present with acute, periodic, short-lived exacerbations of their symptomatology. Drug abuse is a common cause of confusional episodes.

Non-epileptic Staring Spells, Childhood Preoccupation and Daydreaming [52,55,112-114]

Staring spells are a frequent epileptic or non-epileptic manifestation.[52]

Non-epileptic staring spells are at the borderline of the PNEPEs and are more accurately described as (normal) episodes of behavioural inattention that are misinterpreted by an over-vigilant adult.[55] Children frequently experience these benign non-epileptic staring spells, and this 'over-vigilance' is particularly likely to occur when the child also has or has had seizures.

Non-epileptic staring spells, especially in younger children, can take the form of prolonged staring without other features or as inattentiveness with the eyes closed.[52]

The main features that suggest non-epileptic events include:[113]

- The events do not interrupt play
- They are first noticed by a professional such as a schoolteacher, speech therapist, occupational therapist or physician (rather than by a parent)
- The staring spell is 'interruptable' by external stimuli.

Factors associated with an epileptic aetiology include twitches of the arms or legs, loss of urine and upwards eye movement.[113]

Diagnostic Clues for Staring

During a spell of unresponsiveness, documenting an increase in heart rate of more than 30% over baseline has a positive predictive value of 97% in favour of an epileptic event rather than a PNEPE.[53]

Preoccupation implies that the person is concentrating on something tangible and identifiable, such as a television program or an arithmetical calculation.

Daydreaming implies the person is concentrating on something in his or her mind and usually occurs when the child is obviously bored. In both, the child stares ahead, seemingly blankly, and is more or less unresponsive. Colour changes, myoclonic phenomena and changes in muscle tone do not happen. However, automatisms may occur. Usually the child drifts in and out of the attack, although some may 'snap out' of it. In nearly all cases, the episodes can be interrupted.

Inattention or daydreaming was the final diagnosis in 10% of children and adolescents with PNEPEs assessed in an epilepsy monitoring unit.[115]

Daydreams and childhood preoccupations are especially difficult to differentiate from atypical absences in children with learning difficulties; the tendency for the child to drift in and out of the attack may be very similar. The circumstances of when the attacks occur may help.

NEPEs Occurring During Sleep and Sleep Disorders[116-122]

6

Sleep and the epilepsies have reciprocal relationships.[123-129] Sleep accentuates certain types of epileptic seizures, some of which exclusively occur during sleep (nocturnal epilepsy),[130] as well as certain types of epileptiform EEG abnormalities (e.g. benign focal spikes of children). Conversely, epileptic seizures adversely affect sleep quality and architecture.

Some patients with nocturnal seizures become aware of an epileptic seizure because of its adverse effects through injury or post-ictal manifestations. Symptoms such as tongue biting, newly onset bedwetting, unexplained body bruises, confusion or joint dislocations, alone but particularly in combination, discovered upon awakening are highly suggestive of GTCSs. These symptoms may be the reason for why patients first seek medical attention.

Paroxysmal sleep disorders are abnormal episodic phenomena occurring during sleep. The widespread utilisation of videopolysomnography has contributed to the identification of a variety of previously unrecognised sleep disorders and to the better characterisation of already known clinical entities. Diagnosis is made on the basis of medical history and confirmed with videopolysomnography. Treatment is successful in the majority of cases.

Paroxysmal sleep disorders can cause injuries, psychological distress and other deficits from frequent sleep interruption. They may be misdiagnosed and inappropriately treated as epileptic seizures or psychiatric disorders because of sometimes bizarre and hazardous manifestations. Diagnosis is further complicated by the fact that medical and psychiatric disorders and various medications can precipitate or aggravate parasomnias.[131] Misdiagnosis is more likely in children and the elderly.

Classification of Sleep Disorders

According to DSM-IV, sleep disorders may be either *primary* (unrelated to any other disorder – medical or psychological) or *secondary* (the result of physical illness, psychological disorders, or drug or alcohol use).[51]

The primary sleep disorders are categorised as:
- Dyssomnias, which pertain to the amount, quality or timing of sleep
- Parasomnias, which pertain to abnormal behavioural or physiological events that occur during sleep.

C.P. Panayiotopoulos, *Imitators of Epileptic Seizures*, DOI 10.1007/978-1-4471-4023-8_6, © Springer-Verlag London 2012

Dyssomnias include primary insomnia (i.e. sleep-onset insomnia, sleep-maintenance insomnia and terminal insomnia), primary hypersomnia, narcolepsy, breathing-related sleep disorder (sleep apnoea) and circadian rhythm sleep disorder (delayed sleep phase type, jet lag type, shift work type and unspecified type).

Parasomnias are undesirable physical phenomena accompanying sleep that involve skeletal muscle activity or autonomic nervous system changes, or both.[132] Parasomnias include nightmare, sleep terror, sleep walking disorder and many others not listed in the DSM-IV that are detailed in this section.

Parasomnias are grouped into four different categories according to the sleep-state during which they usually occur:
1. Arising from deep sleep (stage III/IV sleep)
2. Associated with REM sleep
3. Sleep–wake transition
4. Other parasomnias non-state sleep-dependent.

Sleep-Related Non-epileptic Movement Disorders[118]

Hypnagogic Myoclonic Jerks (Sleep Starts)

When dropping off to sleep at night one may occasionally experience a sudden, momentarily rather alarming jerk of the whole or a part of the body, sometimes accompanied by a vivid sensory experience… The jerks seem to occur, with widely varying frequencies, in nearly every normal person.

Ian Oswald[133]

Sleep starts (synonyms: *hypnic jerks, hypnagogic jerks, and predormital myoclonus*) are normal phenomena occurring only at the onset of sleep. They usually manifest with jerks of the body, but legs are more likely to be affected than arms. A sharp cry may also occur and there may be concomitant flashes of sensory manifestations; visual hallucinations or dreams, and a feeling of falling.

The frequency and intensity of sleep starts vary. They may be single jerks but more often occur in clusters. They sometimes are very frequent, intense and repetitive, and may cause bruises of the feet by being kicked against the bed, or lead to a bed partner being hurt. This may prevent the individuals from falling asleep, although sometimes it is only the bed partner who experiences these effects. In most people, they only occur from time to time.

Sleep starts affect all ages and both men and women. Adults are more likely to complain about frequent or intense jerks.

Sleep starts are often exacerbated by fatigue, emotional stress, sleep deprivation and high intake of caffeine or other stimulants.

> ### Useful Clinical Note
>
> The significance of hypnagogic jerks in history-taking for epileptic seizures and particularly JME
>
> Patients and witnesses do not usually report myoclonic jerks. The yield of detected myoclonic jerks increases significantly with a physical demonstration of myoclonic jerks (videos may also be very useful). If hypnagogic jerks are reported then it is certain that the concept of myoclonic jerks has been understood.

Nocturnal Myoclonus[134]

Nocturnal myoclonus and nocturnal myoclonic activity is slightly higher in men than in women and correlates with increasing age. Myoclonic activity occurs most frequently during stage II of sleep. The resulting sleep disturbance is usually minimal. Only about 10% of the events relate to EEG arousals.[134]

Fragmentary Hypnic Myoclonus[135-137]

Excessive fragmentary hypnic myoclonus of sleep consists of high amounts of brief twitch-like movements occurring asynchronously and asymmetrically throughout the body, limbs and face. It occurs in all stages of sleep but with a somewhat lower frequency in slow-wave sleep and a significantly lower rate in the first hour after onset compared to later hours. Almost all patients are male. It also occurs in association with other sleep disorders such as periodic limb movements, narcolepsy, intermittent hypersomnia and rarely insomnia.

Propriospinal Myoclonus[138-140]

This consists of recurrent axial jerks or unpleasant sensorimotor symptoms that occur in drowsiness and often prevent sleep. The jerks are slower and more focal than the sleep starts. Propriospinal myoclonus is rarely caused by spinal cord disease.

Benign Neonatal Sleep Myoclonus

Benign neonatal sleep myoclonus is described in chapter 4.

Facio-mandibular Myoclonus[118,141]

Facio-mandibular myoclonus during sleep may cause nocturnal tongue biting and bleeding, which may lead to suspicions of nocturnal GTCS. Electromyography (EMG) activity starts in the masseters and spreads to orbicularis oris and oculi muscles. It mimics sleep bruxism and may be familial.

Restless Legs Syndrome and Periodic Limb Movement Disorder[142-145]

Restless legs syndrome and the periodic limb movement disorder are distinguishable but overlapping diseases. Both feature periodic nocturnal involuntary limb movements that can cause sleep disruption, but each has distinct clinical features that are relevant to the diagnosis and management of the patient.

Periodic limb movements of sleep manifest with brief 0.5–5 s repetitive flexions of the extremities and occur at regular intervals of 10–60 s or in clusters over many minutes which progressively decline throughout the night. They often lead to brief arousals or repeated full awakenings. They can occur as an isolated phenomenon, but are frequently part of the restless legs syndrome or other sleep disorders, although they also occur in normal individuals. They are age related; they occur in less than 1% of young adults and nearly half of the elderly population.

Restless legs syndrome is a sensorimotor disorder that occurs in 1–5% of the population.[146,147] Manifestations mainly consist of unpleasant sensations experienced predominantly in the legs and rarely in the arms. The symptoms occur only at rest and become more pronounced in the evening or at night. In addition, the patients suffer from a strong urge to move the limbs, typically manifested by walking around, which leads to complete but only temporary relief of the symptoms. Most of the patients have periodic limb movements during sleep and relaxed wakefulness. Pharmacological treatments are mainly with dopamine agonists and benzodiazepines.

Rhythmic Movements in Sleep

Rhythmic movements in sleep, also known as jactatio capitis nocturna, may be the same disorder as 'rhythmic behavioural movements'. Rhythmic movements such as head banging or body rocking occur just before sleep onset and persist into light sleep. Rhythmic movements are repeated about every 2 s in long clusters and may be associated with chanting or other vocalisations. This is more common in children, especially infants, but may persist into adulthood.

Children and patients with learning disabilities often exhibit body rocking when awake or asleep. Patients with daytime dyskinesias may occasionally exhibit similar movements during overnight sleep, usually in the setting of brief arousals.

Sleepwalking and Night Terrors[119,148,149]

Sleepwalking (somnambulism) and night terrors (pavor nocturnus) are part of the same nosologic continuum caused by a sudden partial arousal from stage III and IV of NREM sleep (*NREM arousal parasomnias*). They usually occur during the first episode of slow-wave sleep, within the first 2 hours of sleep onset and the timing is often stereotyped. They are characterised by agitation and unresponsiveness to external stimuli. They are usually brief, lasting for 1 or 2 min but may also go on for much longer. Patients are unable to fully awaken, are difficult to comfort and have no memory of the event the next day. The episodes seem to occur in cycles. They may happen every night for several weeks and then disappear for months.

In *pavor nocturnus* the patient manifests intense fright with screaming and moaning together with marked tachycardia, rapid respiration and sweating.

In *somnabulism*, the patient walks around, often performing complex automatic activities. Injuries and occasionally death may occur. Brief, abortive episodes are the most common, involving sitting up in bed with fidgeting and shuffling, as seen with the complex focal seizures.

EEG during these events shows a mixture of slow and alpha activity.[150]

Benign forms of NREM arousal parasomnias have high prevalence of around 10–15% of the population; they occur frequently in childhood and attenuate in adolescence. They can persist into or begin in adulthood with more severe and persisting forms.

Sleepwalking and night terrors may be genetically determined in children while adults show high levels of psychopathology. Additional sleep disorders include sleep-disordered breathing and restless legs syndrome.[149]

Attacks may be eliminated by passively awakening the patient just prior to the habitual time of the events. Trying to awaken the patient during the attacks is pointless.

Night Terrors Are Not Nightmares

Night terrors are stage III or IV NREM disturbances and there are no dreams.
Nightmares occur during, and are the result of, a dream in REM sleep. The sleeper retains a vivid memory of the dream.

Sleep talking is another parasomnia that may be confused with complex focal seizures. Episodes are usually brief, infrequent and may be spontaneous or induced by conversation.

Paroxysmal Nocturnal Dystonia (Hypnogenic Paroxysmal Dystonia)

This is frontal lobe epilepsy of the supplementary motor area and not a sleep disorder.

Sleep-Related Non-epileptic Behavioural and Other Disorders

Sleep Drunkenness[151,152]

'Sleep drunkenness' refers to a failure of attaining full alertness after awakening, usually from deep sleep. The patient appears disorientated, ataxic, dysarthric and may manifest with complex automatic, sometimes aggressive and homicidal, behaviours, as with narcolepsy. This mainly occurs in patients with hypersomnia or after severe sleep deprivation. It may be misdiagnosed as post-ictal confusion or focal complex seizure.

Bruxism[153-156]

Bruxism (teeth grinding and clenching) occurs at any sleep stage but mainly in stage II of NREM sleep. It may also occur during the daytime. It is common in children, especially those with learning disabilities, and psychiatric patients. Dental occlusive appliances are usually an effective treatment. Episodes of bruxism are usually more prolonged and more frequent than focal seizures, and there are no associated features of other motor phenomena, vocalisation or confusional arousal.

Catathrenia (Nocturnal Expiratory Groaning)

This is a rare form of parasomnia of exclusively expiratory groaning during sleep that occurs in clusters of approximately 30 s each. It happens in young people during the second part of the night in REM and stage II of NREM sleep.[157]

Nocturnal Enuresis

Nocturnal enuresis is a very common problem in children and has varying aetiologies.[158] A genetic component is likely. For the idiopathic (primary) nocturnal enuresis there may be two subtypes: those with a functional bladder disorder and those with a maturational delay in nocturnal arginine-vasopressin secretion. Whether in some children nocturnal enuresis is a sleep disorder has been debated.

REM Sleep Behaviour Disorder[159-162]

REM sleep behaviour disorder (RBD) manifests with attacks of vigorous and often dangerous motor activity in response to vivid dreaming in association with intermittent loss of REM sleep skeletal muscle atonia. The patients act out their dreams.

RBD is more prevalent in elderly (mean age 60 years) males (87%) but is also reported in children with autism.[163] Its prevalence in the general population is estimated to be around 0.5%.[161] RBD may be idiopathic (60%) or strongly associated with alpha-synucleinopathies,[161] often heralding the clinical onset of neurodegenerative disease, especially Parkinson's disease, multiple system atrophy and dementia with Lewy bodies. A third of patients injure themselves and two-thirds assault their bed partners. Dream content mostly involves aggressiveness,[160] usually as a defence mechanism against attack.[159]

EEG may show coincidental inter-ictal epileptiform activity of sporadic, frontotemporal sharp waves in a quarter of patients.[164] This may also occur in REM sleep, although rarely. Such EEG abnormalities may reinforce an erroneous diagnosis of nocturnal focal seizures.

Neuroimaging is unlikely to reveal underlying disorders not suspected clinically. Small doses of clonazepam 0.5–1 mg (or melatonin as an alternative) at bedtime are highly effective.[162]

Hypermotor epileptic seizures may be mistaken for RBD. However, the lack of dream recall, the stereotyped movements and occasional SGTCS of hypermotor seizures are useful as distinguishing features.

Sleep-Related Eating Disorder[165]

Some patients have abnormal compulsory nocturnal eating episodes that may be associated with sleepwalking, somniloquy, restless legs syndrome and periodic limb movements during sleep. Eating always occurs after complete awakenings from NREM sleep and exceptionally from REM sleep. During the eating episodes patients are fully alert and EEG shows alpha activity. Most patients manifest with recurring chewing and swallowing movements (resembling the rhythmic masticatory-muscle activity in patients with bruxism) during sleep, which in half of the events is associated with EEG arousals.[165]

Sudden Infant Death Syndrome (Cot Death)[166]

Sudden and unexpected death of an infant during sleep and without postmortem abnormal findings is a rare and tragic event. It occurs mainly between 10 and 12 weeks of age. An epileptic seizure may sometimes be the actual cause.

Narcolepsy[119,167-175]

Narcolepsy is a sleep disorder with frequent episodes of REM-sleep that occur inappropriately before NREM sleep. In wakefulness, REM periods or fragments of REM occur throughout the day.

Demographic Data

Narcolepsy usually begins in childhood[173] with a higher incidence in adolescence (16–30 years). Prevalence is 0.05% in Caucasians and three times higher in Japanese.

Clinical Manifestations

Narcolepsy manifests with the tetrad of:

1. *Hypersomnia* (*excessive and irresistible daytime sleepiness*), which includes the following: daytime sleep attacks, which may occur with or without warning; persistent drowsiness, which may continue for prolonged periods of time; and 'microsleeps', or fleeting moments of sleep. Sleep attacks may happen while standing, eating, driving or during a conversation. Episodes of automatic behaviour (performing a task without conscious awareness of doing it) and amnesia are common, as in all other cases of hypersomnia. Their duration ranges from seconds to 15–30 min and they usually end with a sudden burst of irrelevant words.
2. *Cataplexy*, which consists of a sudden loss of voluntary muscle control, triggered by strong emotions such as laughter, surprise, fear or anger. The attacks mainly affect facial and leg muscles (e.g. sagging, nodding, buckling knees, muddled speech), they may be experienced as mild weakness only

and can last for seconds or 15–30 min. Total body collapse may occur with full preservation of consciousness. Cataplexy is sometimes instantaneous with no time to prepare for safety, and thus serious injury can occur.

3. *Sleep paralysis*, which is a brief (seconds to usually 10 min), temporary inability to move that occurs on falling asleep (hypnagogic) and less often on awakening.

Cataplexy and sleep paralysis are related to the muscle atonia of REM.

4. *Hallucinations*, which appear as vivid, realistic, often frightening 'dreams of REM' occur upon falling asleep (hypnagogic) and less often upon awakening. Visual hallucinations are more common than auditory, vestibular or somatosensory hallucinations. They may occur together or precede sleep paralysis.

The patients are fully aware of cataplexy, sleep paralysis and hallucinations.

All patients with narcolepsy have hypersomnia but only around 70% also develop cataplexy; sleep paralysis and hypnagogic hallucination occur in a third.

The clinical picture of narcolepsy is further complicated by intense fatigue, memory problems and visual problems, frequent sleep arousals and other sleep disorders, as well as the psychological and social consequences of having narcolepsy.

Aetiology[175]

Narcolepsy is familial in 10% of cases. Mutations in the region of chromosome 6 controlling the HLA antigen immune complex are found in 90–100% of patients, but these also occur in as many as 50% of people without narcolepsy. Narcolepsy has been attributed to a deficiency of the peptide neurotransmitter hypocretin produced in the hypothalamus. A dog model of narcolepsy exhibits a mutation on chromosome 12 that disrupts the processing of hypocretin. No such mutations were found in human narcolepsy but hypocretin levels are profoundly depressed in cerebrospinal fluid (CSF) and a specific reduction in hypocretin-containing neurones has been described. One hypothesis concerning the pathophysiology of narcolepsy proposes that the HLA subtype resulting from the mutation on chromosome 6 increases the susceptibility of hypocretin-containing brain neurones to immune attack. Because hypocretin may normally participate in the maintenance of wakefulness, the loss of neurones that release this peptide might allow inappropriate occurrence of REM sleep in contrast to its normal cyclic appearance after NREM sleep.

Diagnostic Procedures

Overnight polysomnography is often diagnostic and may also reveal other underlying sleep disorders. The multiple sleep latency test (MSLT) measures sleep onset and how quickly REM sleep occurs. A blood genetic test has been developed that measures certain antigens often found in people who have a predisposition to narcolepsy. Positive results suggest but do not prove narcolepsy.

Differential Diagnosis

Narcolepsy should be differentiated from other causes of hypersomnia. Cataplexy is almost unique to narcolepsy but the presence of cataplexy is not required for a diagnosis of narcolepsy.

Cataplectic attacks may be misdiagnosed as atonic seizures, other types of epileptic falls or syncope. Episodes of automatic behaviour may be confused with complex focal seizures.

Isolated episodes of sleep paralysis, cataplectic attacks and hallucinations can occur frequently in normal people.

Prognosis

Narcolepsy is a lifelong disorder with no signs of remission or improvement.

Management[167,174]

Modafinil is the first-line pharmacological treatment of excessive daytime sleepiness and irresistible episodes of sleep in association with behavioural measures. Sodium oxybate is the first-line treatment of cataplexy and appears to also have a beneficial effect on excessive daytime sleepiness and disturbed nocturnal sleep.

Sleep Apnoea

Patients with sleep apnoea usually present with day-time hypersomnia, and apnoeic episodes may cause episodic grunting, flailing about or other restless activity that appears to mimic nocturnal epilepsy. Occasionally the resultant hypoxia leads itself to symptomatic epileptic seizures.

Apnoeic attacks in neonates, whether while awake or asleep, are difficult to differentiate from epileptic seizures.

Sleep Disorders in the Elderly

Sleep undergoes significant changes with ageing and these are so profound that it is difficult to separate normal from disease.[176] Sleep disorders are estimated to affect nearly 50% of older individuals. These are mostly sleep-disordered breathing, periodic limb movements in sleep and restless legs syndrome, morning headaches, circadian rhythm disorders, excessive daytime sleepiness, RBD, obstructive sleep apnoea and insomnia.[177]

Subjective Non-epileptic Paroxysmal Symptoms Imitating Simple Focal Seizures

7

Visual, Auditory, Somatosensory, Olfactory, Gustatory and Autonomic Paroxysmal Symptoms Imitating Simple Focal Seizures[178]

There is a galaxy of subjective paroxysmal symptoms that may imitate, and in some cases are identical to, those occurring in simple focal epileptic seizures. These are subjective sensations, simple or complex visual hallucinations or illusions that may be:

- Normal experiences of healthy people
- Caused by a variety of abnormalities located in the peripheral sensory organs or in the CNS
- Of multiple aetiologies (drugs or various brain, psychiatric and systemic disorders)

Thus, the differential diagnosis of these paroxysmal symptoms is extensive, spanning numerous normal phenomena, intoxication, and neurological, systemic and psychiatric disorders. Diagnosis is possible and usually straightforward if the symptoms are analysed and synthesised in a meaningful manner with regard to their various parameters and characteristics (quality, quantity, time and duration of appearance), development, stereotype, recurrence, precipitating factors, other concurrent symptoms, diseases, drug use, age and so forth. Long-term recurrent isolated subjective sensations without any other symptoms are unlikely to be epileptic seizures, because at some time they would have progressed to more apparent ictal seizure manifestations. Visual symptoms of paroxysmal occurrence are probably among the most common imitators of epileptic seizures.[179-183] The example of visual aura of migraine versus visual occipital seizures has been emphasised in chapter 8.

Cyclic Vomiting, Paroxysmal Vertigo and Motion Sickness

Cyclic vomiting syndrome (CVS), paroxysmal vertigo and motion sickness are unlikely to be misdiagnosed as epilepsy. However, some children who are assumed to have CVS or motion sickness may actually be suffering from autonomic seizures or autonomic status epilepticus of Panayiotopoulos syndrome in which emetic symptoms are usually prominent and sometimes occur while, and are probably facilitated by, travelling.[24,184]

C.P. Panayiotopoulos, *Imitators of Epileptic Seizures*,
DOI 10.1007/978-1-4471-4023-8_7, © Springer-Verlag London 2012

Cyclic Vomiting Syndrome[184-187]

CVS has the following characteristics:

- It is specific to childhood (3–9 years)
- Vomiting usually starts in sleep and may last for many hours
- Emetic symptoms are the first to appear but these are often associated with other autonomic manifestations

CVS is an idiopathic non-epileptic disorder of unknown aetiology characterised by periodic clusters of episodic vomiting, often 6–12 times/h. The pattern is stereotypical within individuals and typified by a rapid onset during the night or early morning, rapid denouement and associated symptoms of pallor, lethargy, anorexia, nausea, retching, vomiting, drooling, diarrhoea, abdominal pain and classical headache, photophobia and phonophobia, but rarely visual disturbances. EEG may show only focal slowing at the time of episodes. On rare occasions focal spikes and waves also appear; these may be a coincidental finding because of the high prevalence of functional spikes in children or they may indicate misdiagnosis.

CVS affects young children aged 3–9 years and resolves during adolescence. A third of patients later develop migraine headaches.

Prevalence may be about 2 % of school-aged children, although clinically many may be missed or their symptoms are mild. The vomiting appears to be triggered by a variety of physical and psychological stresses.

The diagnosis of CVS requires exclusionary laboratory testing because it can mimic many surgical, neurological, endocrine, metabolic or renal disorders.

CVS bears considerable similarities to abdominal migraine and to migraine headaches 'though their precise relation and overlap cannot be definitely settled until validated laboratory markers become available'.[185]

The pathogenesis of CVS is unknown but there are now several tenable mechanisms such as migraine, metabolic, neuroendocrine and gastrointestinal.[185] There may also be specific subgroups that have different mechanisms.[185]

CVS is considered to originate in the brain and various mechanisms, probably inter-related, are speculated:

- Corticotrophin-releasing factor, which may be the primary mediator of vomiting in CVS[186]
- Mitochondrial DNA mutations and disordered respiratory chain function[186]
- Defects in the regulation of cellular mechanisms such as cAMP or ion channels in cells at critical locations in the emetic pathway (e.g. nucleus tractus solitarius, area postrema)
- Defects in intrinsic pathways (e.g. opioid neurones) that may modulate the brain-stem emetic mechanisms[187]

Treatment options are improving at present and serotonergic agents have shown the most promise.

Benign Positional Paroxysmal Vertigo

Benign positional paroxysmal vertigo is the most frequent cause of vertigo in adults and manifests with brief episodes of spinning vertigo precipitated by movement such as bending over, turning in bed, looking up or driving. Nausea can be a prominent feature or absent. Attacks may be very frequent and the disorder, although benign, may be disabling. It is a disease of the semicircular canal and occurs when freely floating otoconia enter one or more of the semi-circular canals and move under the influence of gravity. It is rarely observed in individuals younger than 35 years without a history of antecedent head trauma. The Epley manoeuvre for repositioning the displaced otoconia is a simple technique that often has therapeutic efficacy.

Benign Paroxysmal Vertigo of Childhood

Benign paroxysmal vertigo of childhood is the most common cause of vertigo in children without any detectable ear disease or hearing loss. It manifests with typical vestibular attack including nystagmus, nausea, vomiting and dia-phoresis. The age at onset is usually 1–5 years old. It has been related to migraine and some experts consider it as a precursor of migraine.

Motion Sickness

Motion sickness is a common response to real and perceived movement in the environment.[188-192] It occurs while travelling via any form of transport. Children aged between 4 and 10 years are particularly vulnerable. Girls are more susceptible than boys.

Symptoms begin with epigastric discomfort, which is usually accompanied by increased salivation, eructation and a feeling of bodily warmth. With sustained exposure to the triggering stimulus, symptoms progress to nausea, pallor, sweating and, eventually, retching or vomiting. A variant of motion sickness may exist that lacks gastrointestinal complaints and is instead char-acterised by drowsiness, headache, apathy, depression and generalised discomfort.

Migraine, Migralepsy, Basilar Migraine with EEG Occipital Paroxysms and Diagnostic Errors

8

Migraine with aura may be misdiagnosed as epilepsy but, far more frequently, epileptic seizures are misdiagnosed as migraine.[193-195] As a result, visual occipital lobe seizures (misdiagnosed as visual aura of migraine and SGTCSs) are erroneously attributed to the migraine effect on the brain (hence the inappropriate term 'migralepsy').[196]

Migraine and epilepsy are the most common neurological disorders. Prevalence of migraine is probably around 6% for men and three times more frequent in women. Epilepsy is around 0.5% and equally affects men and women. If a relationship existed between them, this would be obvious in our everyday neurological practice. It would not be revealed only through obscure and complicated cases with bizarre symptomatology. It would be simple and common. It is not. The problem is that occipital seizures are not appropriately differentiated from migraine and, therefore, they are often erroneously diagnosed as migraine.

Seizures may be triggered by a migrainous event or caused by a migraine–stroke but this is rare. There should be no doubt that cerebral infarcts due to severe migraine can be responsible for symptomatic seizures. Also, there should be no reason why epileptic seizures, so vulnerable to extrinsic and intrinsic precipitating factors, could not also be susceptible to cortical changes introduced by migraine. Thus a migrainous attack may also be able to trigger epileptic seizures in susceptible individuals. However, both these cases are rare. In my opinion, the most common reason for their association is through the coincidence of two of the most common neurological disorders and an erroneous interpretation of epileptic seizures as migraine or, less often, *vice versa*. The emerging and more realistic concept of occipital seizures triggering migrainous headache needs consideration and exploration. More importantly, patients with daily visual seizures that may progress to convulsions merit a precise diagnosis and appropriate treatment probably with carbamazepine. Most of these patients with visual seizures are misdiagnosed as migraine with aura, basilar migraine, acephalgic migraine or migralepsy simply because physicians are not properly informed of differential diagnostic criteria. As a result, diagnosis, appropriate investigations and treatment may be delayed for years. There are numerous published reports of such a misdiagnosis. Such

C.P. Panayiotopoulos, *Imitators of Epileptic Seizures*,
DOI 10.1007/978-1-4471-4023-8_8, © Springer-Verlag London 2012

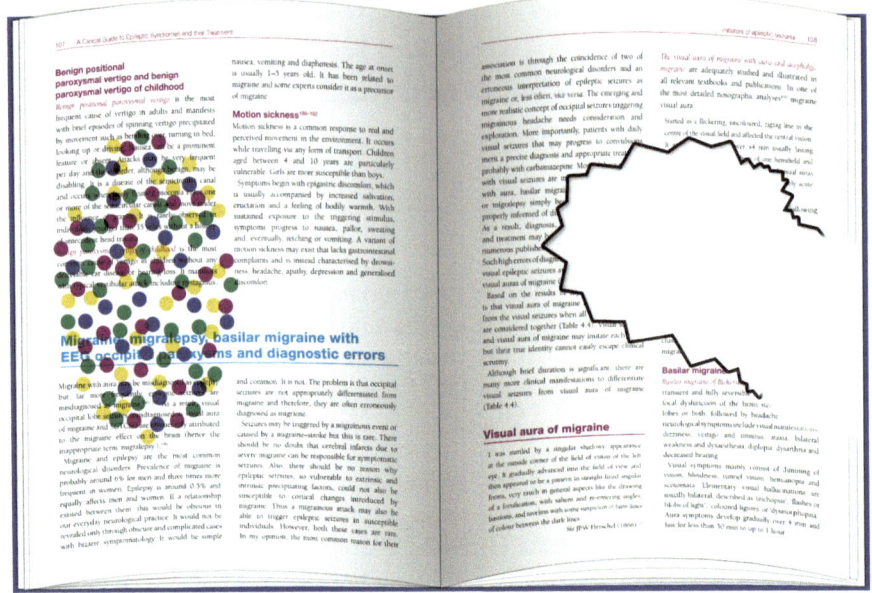

Fig. 8.1 Schematic illustration of elementary visual hallucinations of visual occipital lobe epileptic seizures (*left*) and visual aura of migraine (*right*) (Adapted with permission from Panayiotopoulos[196])

high errors of diagnosis are unjustifiable because visual epileptic seizures are distinctly different from visual auras of migraine (Fig. 8.1).[194,195]

Based on the results of my studies, my thesis is that visual aura of migraine is entirely different from the visual seizures when all their components are considered together (Table 8.1). Visual seizures and visual aura of migraine may imitate each other but their true identity cannot easily escape clinical scrutiny.

Although brief duration is significant, there are many more clinical manifestations to differentiate visual seizures from visual aura of migraine (Table 8.1).

Visual Aura of Migraine

I was startled by a singular shadowy appearance at the outside corner of the field of vision of the left eye. It gradually advanced into the field of view and then appeared to be a pattern in straight-lined angular forms, very much in general aspects like the drawing of a fortification, with salient and re-entering angles, bastions, and ravelins with some suspicion of faint lines of colour between the dark lines.

Sir JFW Herschel[197]

	Occipital epilepsy	Migraine with aura	Basilar migraine
Visual hallucinations			
Duration for seconds to 1 min	Exclusive	None	None
Duration for 1–3 min	Frequent	Rare	Rare
Duration for 4–30 min	Rare	As a rule	As a rule
Daily in frequency	As a rule	Rare	None
Mainly coloured circular patterns	As a rule	Rare	Exceptional
Mainly achromatic or black and white linear patterns	Exceptional	As a rule	Rare
Moving to the opposite side of the visual field	Exclusive	None	None
Expanding from the centre to the periphery of a visual hemifield	Rare	As a rule	Frequent
Evolving to blindness	Rare	Rare	As a rule
Evolving to tonic deviation of eyes	Exclusive	None	None
Evolving to impairment of consciousness without convulsions	Frequent	Rare	Frequent
Evolving to impairment of consciousness with convulsions	Frequent	Exceptional	Rare
Associated with post-ictal/post-critical headache	Frequent	As a rule	Frequent
Blindness and hemianopia			
Without other preceding or following symptoms	Frequent	None	Frequent
Brain-stem symptoms	None	None	Exclusive
Post-ictal/post-critical vomiting	Rare	Frequent	Frequent
Post-ictal/post-critical severe headache	Frequent	As a rule	Frequent

Modified with permission from Panayiotopoulos[195]

Table 8.1 Differential diagnosis of occipital seizures from migraine with aura or basilar migraine

The visual aura of migraine with aura and acephalgic migraine are adequately studied and illustrated in all relevant textbooks and publications. In one of the most detailed nosographic analyses[198] migraine visual aura:

> *Started as a flickering, uncoloured, zigzag line in the centre of the visual field and affected the central vision. It gradually progressed over >4 min usually lasting <30 min towards the periphery of one hemifield and often left a scotoma. The total duration of visual auras was 60 min. Only four patients had exclusively acute onset visual aura.[198]*

Furthermore, migraine visual aura has the following characteristics:

- It rarely has a daily frequency
- Non-visual ictal occipital symptoms such as eye and head deviation, and eyelid repetitive closures do not occur
- It is debatable and probably exceptional to progress to non-visual epileptic seizures.

Less typical features of migraine visual aura such as spots, circles and beads with or without colours may be experienced during the migraine visual aura but usually they are not dominant. More importantly, clustering of other symptoms, as above, betray their migraine nature.

Basilar Migraine

Basilar migraine of Bickerstaff[199,200] is characterised by transient and fully reversible symptoms, indicating focal dysfunction of the brain stem, the occipital lobes or both, followed by headache.[201] Common neurological symptoms include visual manifestations, dizziness, vertigo and tinnitus, ataxia, bilateral weakness and dysaesthesia, diplopia, dysarthria and decreased hearing.

Visual symptoms mainly consist of dimming of vision, blindness, tunnel vision, hemianopia and scotomata. Elementary visual hallucinations are usually bilateral, described as 'teichopsia', 'flashes or blobs of light', 'coloured figures' or 'dysmorphopsia'. Aura symptoms develop gradually over 4 min and last for less than 30 min to up to 1 h.

Impairment or loss of consciousness without convulsions may occur in a quarter of patients between the aura and the headache phase.

> *The loss of consciousness is described as curiously slow in onset – never abrupt, and never causing the patient to fall or to be injured. A dreamlike state sometimes precedes impairment of consciousness. The degree of impairment of consciousness was never profound but the patients were never unrousable; on vigorous stimulation they could be aroused to co-operate but they returned to unconsciousness when the stimulation ceased.[200]*

Attacks of basilar migraine are usually infrequent and over the years they may cease or become replaced by common migraine with or without aura.[201]

Migralepsy

Migralepsy – migra(ine) and (epi)lepsy – is a term used to denote 'a seizure that may be a composite of symptoms encountered in epilepsy and migraine'.[202,203] *Intercalated seizures* denote epileptic seizures that occur between the migrainous aura and the headache phase of migraine.[204]

I would discourage the use of the term migralepsy. According to a recent review, most reported cases of so-called migralepsy are likely to be genuine occipital seizures imitating migraine aura.[194,195] Of the most influential cases that I have detailed,[194,195] two of the three 'migralepsy' patients,[202] one 'basilar migraine and epilepsy case'[205] and one 'juvenile migraine with epilepsy' boy,[206] all had symptoms of visual seizures – as defined in this booklet – that were interpreted as migraine aura. The 'juvenile migraine' patient of Barlow[206] with symptomatic occipital epilepsy may be indicative:

This boy at age 13 years 'While ski-ing... saw blue to the right associated with blurred vision that lasted for a few seconds' after which he vomited, became confused for 30 min, followed by a severe throbbing headache. Subsequently he had occasional 'episodes of similar visual disturbance' diagnosed as juvenile migraine successfully treated with phenytoin. An arteriovenous malformation was found in the left occipital lobe. 'Visual scotomata accompanied by flashing lights that only occasionally were followed by headache' continued post-operatively.

None of the 1550 patients I have studied had any evidence of seizures developing from migraine aura, although this was often the initial erroneous diagnosis on referral.[195] Conversely, post-ictal headache and other migraine-like symptoms frequently occurred after occipital seizures. However, an incontrovertible diagnosis may be difficult in some equivocal cases:

A 38-year-old man, who while working with the computer, saw flashing light in between his eyes. They were moving for a few centimetres upwards and to the right repetitively. Gradually, the intensity of the light and the area increased in the next 30 min obscuring his vision. This ended with a GTCS as he was entering the examination room of his general practitioner where he went walking for help. He had never experienced similar symptoms, seizures or migraine in the past. MRI was normal. EEG showed minor non-specific abnormalities.

Visual Seizures

They commenced with the appearance of several small spheres, white in the centre with an intermediate zone of blue and outside this a ring of red, immediately to the left of the point at which the patient gazed; from here they moved either at a uniform rate or in jerks to the left and downwards... In all attacks the eyes deviated towards the left and the head turned in the same direction as soon as the visual spectra appeared.

G. Holmes[207]

The elementary hallucinations of visual epileptic seizures are detailed in the relevant section of occipital lobe epilepsy (see Chapter 15, page 474, and Table 8.1).[194,195] Briefly, elementary visual hallucinations of visual seizures are mainly coloured and circular, develop fast (within seconds) and are of brief duration (Fig. 8.1). They often appear in the periphery of a temporal visual hemifield, becoming larger and multiplying in the course of the seizure, frequently moving horizontally towards the other side. They are fundamentally different to the visual aura of migraine with which they are often mistaken.[194,195,208]

Differentiating Visual Seizures from Migraine

The misdiagnosis of visual seizures as migraine appears to be high, although their differentiation should not be difficult.[193-196] Occipital seizures manifesting with elementary visual hallucinations, blindness and headache, alone or in combination, may imitate migraine, which is the reason why they are often mistaken for migraine with aura, acephalgic or basilar migraine (Table 8.1 and Fig. 8.1)[194,195] Even lesional occipital epilepsy is often misdiagnosed as migraine and, on many occasions, visual seizures are considered as a visual aura of migraine, thus limiting their prognostic significance with regard to the continuation of treatment.[195] The following are quotes from medical referrals of patients with visual seizures:

> *This patient has visual migraine-like disturbances, such as teichopsias.*
> *Scintillating scotoma or sparkling scotoma of migraine.*
> *Migrainous aura before the fit.*

Diagnostic Tips

Factors contributing to error in the diagnosis of visual seizures

The major contributory factor to error is that the description of visual hallucinations is often abbreviated in terms such as fortification spectrum, teichopsia, scintillating scotoma, phosphenes and their variations.[208] Their meaning does not always represent the actual descriptions, which should be meticulously requested. Erroneously, they are frequently unquestionably equated with migraine.

Diagnostic Tips

As a rule, brief (<1 min), elementary visual hallucinations that develop rapidly within seconds, with coloured and circular patterns and daily frequency are probably pathognomonic of visual seizures, despite the severe headache and vomiting that may follow. EEGs may be normal, show non-specific abnormalities, or reveal slow focal or occipital spikes. A high-resolution MRI is mandatory because it may detect a structural lesion requiring early attention and management.

There are two main reasons that visual seizures are misdiagnosed as migraine.[193-195] First, visual seizures are not examined in a comprehensive manner; instead they are abbreviated to terms such as 'scintillating scotoma' or 'teichopsia', which often do not represent the actual description of the patients. Second, their differential diagnostic criteria have only recently been adequately studied and addressed.[194,195,208] The diagnosis of visual seizures may comfortably rely on clinical criteria only; other investigative procedures are essential, but even ictal EEG may not identify a third or more of cases.

Misconceptions

There is a misconception that there is a syndrome of 'basilar migraine with EEG occipital paroxysms', which is perpetuated in every relevant publication and textbook to date. Retrospective analysis of cases described as 'basilar migraine with occipital paroxysms'[209-212] showed that these patients genuinely suffer from idiopathic occipital epilepsy.[193,195,212]

Note of Caution

A recent population-based, case–control study concluded that children with migraine with aura have a substantial increased risk of developing subsequent epilepsy (odds ratio, 8.1; 95% CI, 2.7–24.3).[213] Migraine without aura did not increase the risk for epilepsy. The diagnosis was made on clinical grounds. However, considering the differential diagnostic problems and the frequency by which epilepsy is misdiagnosed as migraine, I would like to raise this note of caution for such a conclusion and its important consequences.

Appendix

Cerebrovascular NEPEs Imitating Epileptic Seizures

Cerebrovascular disease is a common cause of epileptic seizures, particularly in the elderly. However, with the exception of vertebrobasilar falls and transient ischaemic attacks, cerebrovascular accidents are unlikely to be misdiagnosed as epileptic seizures.

Transient ischaemic attacks are brief episodes of neurological dysfunction caused by focal brain or retinal ischaemia, with clinical symptoms typically lasting less than 1 h, and without evidence of acute infarction. Symptoms are usually negative phenomena of blindness, paresis or other deficits. The difficulty, therefore, in their differentiation from focal seizures arises when positive phenomena such as paraesthesiae occur. Furthermore, transient ischaemic attacks are not usually stereotyped or repeated with the frequency of epileptic seizures, and there are usually associated features to suggest vascular disease.

Falls in vertebrobasilar insufficiency are of sudden onset often with other concurrent features of brain-stem ischaemia such as diplopia, vertigo and bilateral motor-sensory symptoms. They commonly affect elderly people, with evidence of vascular disease and cervical spondylosis. They are usually precipitated by head turning or neck extension resulting in the distortion of vertebral arteries.

C.P. Panayiotopoulos, *Imitators of Epileptic Seizures*,
DOI 10.1007/978-1-4471-4023-8, © Springer-Verlag London 2012

References

1. Crompton DE, Berkovic SF. The borderland of epilepsy: clinical and molecular features of phenomena that mimic epileptic seizures. Lancet Neurol. 2009;8:370–81.
2. Reuber M, Elger CE. Psychogenic nonepileptic seizures: review and update. Epilepsy Behav. 2003;4:205–16.
3. Kaplan PW, Fisher RS, editors. Imitators of epilepsy. 2nd ed. New York: Demos; 2005.
4. Guidelines for Epidemiologic Studies on Epilepsy. Commission on epidemiology and prognosis, international league against epilepsy. Epilepsia. 1993;34:592–6.
5. ILAE Commission Report. The epidemiology of the epilepsies: future directions. International League Against Epilepsy. Epilepsia. 1997;38:614–8.
6. Gates JR. Nonepileptic seizures: classification, coexistence with epilepsy, diagnosis, therapeutic approaches, and consensus. Epilepsy Behav. 2002;3:28–33.
7. National Institute for Health and Clinical Excellence (NICE). The epilepsies: the diagnosis and management of the epilepsies in adults and children in primary and secondary care. www.nice.org.uk/page.aspx?o=227586; 2004. Last accessed 12 Sept 2009.
8. Anonymous. Epilepsy in children: making sense of the diagnostic puzzle. Lancet Neurol. 2005;4:451.
9. Ropper AH, Brown RH. Adam and Victor's principles of neurology. 8th ed. New York: McGraw-Hill; 2005.
10. Panayiotopoulos CP. The epilepsies: seizures, syndromes and management. Oxford: Bladon Medical Publishing; 2005.
11. Panayiotopoulos CP, editor. A practical guide to childhood epilepsies. The educational kit on epilepsies. Oxford: Medicinae; 2006.
12. Panayiotopoulos CP, editor. Idiopathic generalised epilepsies with myoclonic jerks. Oxford: Medicinae; 2007.
13. Chung SS, Gerber P, Kirlin KA. Ictal eye closure is a reliable indicator for psychogenic nonepileptic seizures. Neurology. 2006;66:1730–1.
14. Gastaut H, Broughton R. Epileptic seizures. Clinical and electrographic features, diagnosis and treatment. Springfield: Charles C Thomas; 1972.
15. Donat JF, Wright FS. Clinical imitators of infantile spasms. J Child Neurol. 1992;7:395–9.
16. Caraballo RH, Capovilla G, Vigevano F, Beccaria F, Specchio N, Fejerman N. The spectrum of benign myoclonus of early infancy: clinical and neurophysiologic features in 102 patients. Epilepsia. 2009;50:1176–83.
17. Dalla Bernardina B. Benign myoclonus of early infancy or Fejerman syndrome. Epilepsia. 2009;50:1290–2.
18. Maydell BV, Berenson F, Rothner AD, Wyllie E, Kotagal P. Benign myoclonus of early infancy: an imitator of West's syndrome. J Child Neurol. 2001;16:109–12.
19. Blume WT, Luders HO, Mizrahi E, Tassinari C, van Emde BW, Engel Jr J. Glossary of descriptive terminology for ictal semiology: report of the ILAE task force on classification and terminology. Epilepsia. 2001;42:1212–8.
20. Tassinari CA, Michelucci R, Shigematsu H, Seino M. Atonic and myoclonic-atonic seizures. In: Engel Jr J, Pedley TA, editors. Epilepsy: a comprehensive textbook. 2nd ed. Philadelphia: Lippincott William and Wilkins; 2008. p. 601–9.
21. Tinuper P, Cerullo A, Marini C, Avoni P, Rosati A, Riva R, et al. Epileptic drop attacks in partial epilepsy: clinical features, evolution, and prognosis. J Neurol Neurosurg Psychiatry. 1998;64:231–7.
22. Capovilla G, Rubboli G, Beccaria F, Meregalli S, Veggiotti P, Giambelli PM, et al. Intermittent falls and fecal incontinence as a manifestation of epileptic negative myoclonus in idiopathic partial epilepsy of childhood. Neuropediatrics. 2000;31:273–5.
23. Parry SW, Kenny RA. Drop attacks in older adults: systematic assessment has a high diagnostic yield. J Am Geriatr Soc. 2005;53:74–8.
23a. Panayiotopoulos CP. A clinical guide to epileptic syndromes and their treatment. Revised 2nd edition. London: Springer, 2010.
24. Covanis A. Panayiotopoulos syndrome: a benign childhood autonomic epilepsy frequently imitating encephalitis, syncope, migraine, sleep disorder, or gastroenteritis. Pediatrics. 2006;118:e1237–43.

25. Stephenson JB. Fits and faints. London: MacKeith Press; 1990.
26. Kapoor WN. Syncope. N Engl J Med. 2000;343:1856–62.
27. Brignole M, Alboni P, Benditt D, Bergfeldt L, Blanc JJ, Bloch Thomsen PE, et al. Guidelines on management (diagnosis and treatment) of syncope. Eur Heart J. 2001;22:1256–306.
28. Eiris-Punal J, Rodriguez-Nunez A, Fernandez-Martinez N, Fuster M, Castro-Gago M, Martinon JM. Usefulness of the head-upright tilt test for distinguishing syncope and epilepsy in children. Epilepsia. 2001;42:709–13.
29. Lempert T. Convulsive syncope. In: Gilman S, editor. Medlink neurology. 2009th ed. San Diego: Arbor Publishing Corp; 2009.
30. Schnipper JL, Kapoor WN. Diagnostic evaluation and management of patients with syncope. Med Clin North Am. 2001;85:423–56.
31. Stephenson JB. Anoxic seizures: self-terminating syncopes. Epileptic Disord. 2001;3:3–6.
32. Sheldon R, Rose S, Ritchie D, Connolly SJ, Koshman ML, Lee MA, et al. Historical criteria that distinguish syncope from seizures. J Am Coll Cardiol. 2002;40:142–8.
33. Soteriades ES, Evans JC, Larson MG, Chen MH, Chen L, Benjamin EJ, et al. Incidence and prognosis of syncope. N Engl J Med. 2002;347:878–85.
34. Benditt D, Blanc JJ, Brignole M, Sutton R. Evaluation and treatment of syncope. London: Blackwell Publishing; 2003.
35. McLeod KA. Syncope in childhood. Arch Dis Child. 2003;88:350–3.
36. Britton JW. Syncope and seizures-differential diagnosis and evaluation. Clin Auton Res. 2004;14:148–59.
37. Stephenson JBP, Zuberi S. Nonepileptic seizures and similar phenomena in children and adolescents. In: Kaplan PW, Fisher RS, editors. Imitators of epilepsy. 2nd ed. New York: Demos; 2005. p. 89–109.
38. McKeon A, Vaughan C, Delanty N. Seizure versus syncope. Lancet Neurol. 2006;5:171–80.
39. Zuberi SM, Stephenson JBP. Syncopal and cardiac attacks imitating or provoking epileptic seizures. In: Panayiotopoulos CP, editor. A practical guide to childhood epilepsies, vol. 1. Oxford: Medicinae; 2006. p. 115–22.
40. Lempert T, Bauer M, Schmidt D. Syncope: a videometric analysis of 56 episodes of transient cerebral hypoxia. Ann Neurol. 1994;36:233–7.
41. Benke T, Hochleitner M, Bauer G. Aura phenomena during syncope. Eur Neurol. 1997;37:28–32.
42. Lempert T. Recognizing syncope: pitfalls and surprises. J R Soc Med. 1996;89:372–5.
43. Lempert T, von Brevern M. The eye movements of syncope. Neurology. 1996;46:1086–8.
44. Humm AM, Mathias CJ. Unexplained syncope – is screening for carotid sinus hypersensitivity indicated in all patients aged >40 years? J Neurol Neurosurg Psychiatry. 2006;77:1267–70.
45. Kerr SR, Pearce MS, Brayne C, Davis RJ, Kenny RA. Carotid sinus hypersensitivity in asymptomatic older persons: implications for diagnosis of syncope and falls. Arch Intern Med. 2006;166:515–20.
46. Stephenson J, Breningstall G, Steer C, Kirkpatrick M, Horrocks I, Nechay A, et al. Anoxic-epileptic seizures: home video recordings of epileptic seizures induced by syncopes. Epileptic Disord. 2004;6:15–9.
46a. Koutroumanidis M, Ferrie CD, Valeta T, Sanders S, Michael M, Panayiotopoulos CP. Syncope-like epileptic seizures in panayiotopoulos syndrome. Neurology 2012;(in press).
47. Lesser RP. Psychogenic seizures. Neurology. 1996;46:1499–507.
48. Gumnit RJ. Psychogenic seizures. In: Wyllie E, editor. The treatment of epilepsy: principles and practices. Philadelphia: Lippincott Williams & Wilkins; 2001. p. 699–703.
49. Gates JR, Rowan AJ. Nonepileptic seizures. Boston: Butterworth-Heinemann; 2000.
50. Alper K, Devinsky O, Perrine K, Vazquez B, Luciano D. Psychiatric classification of nonconversion nonepileptic seizures. Arch Neurol. 1995;52:199–201.
51. American Psychiatric Association. Diagnostic and statistical manual of mental disorders. 4th ed, text revision. Washington, DC: American Psychiatric Association; 2000.
52. Carmant L, Kramer U, Holmes GL, Mikati MA, Riviello JJ, Helmers SL. Differential diagnosis of staring spells in children: a video – EEG study. Pediatr Neurol. 1996;14:199–202.
53. Opherk C, Hirsch LJ. Ictal heart rate differentiates epileptic from non-epileptic seizures. Neurology. 2002;58:636–8.
54. Kanner AM, LaFrance Jr WC, Betts T. Psychogenic non-epileptic seizures. In: Engel J Jr J, Pedley TA, editors. Epilepsy: a comprehensive textbook. 2nd ed. Philadelphia: Lippincott William and Wilkins; 2008. p. 2795–810.
55. Benbadis SR. Psychogenic disorders imitating epilepsy. In: Panayiotopoulos CP, editor. A practical guide to childhood epilepsies, vol. 1. Oxford: Medicinae; 2006. p. 133–8.
56. Chabolla DR, Shih JJ. Postictal behaviors associated with psychogenic nonepileptic seizures. Epilepsy Behav. 2006;9:307–11.
57. Howell SJ, Owen L, Chadwick DW. Pseudostatus epilepticus. Q J Med. 1989;71:507–19.
58. Reuber M, Pukrop R, Mitchell AJ, Bauer J, Elger CE. Clinical significance of recurrent psychogenic nonepileptic seizure status. J Neurol. 2003;250:1355–62.

59. Holtkamp M, Othman J, Buchheim K, Meierkord H. Diagnosis of psychogenic nonepileptic status epilepticus in the emergency setting. Neurology. 2006;66:1727–9.
60. Dworetzky BA, Mortati KA, Rossetti AO, Vaccaro B, Nelson A, Bromfield EB. Clinical characteristics of psychogenic nonepileptic seizure status in the long-term monitoring unit. Epilepsy Behav. 2006;9:335–8.
61. de Timary P, Fouchet P, Sylin M, Indriets JP, De Barsy T, Lefebvre A, et al. Non-epileptic seizures: delayed diagnosis in patients presenting with electroencephalographic (EEG) or clinical signs of epileptic seizures. Seizure. 2002;11:193–7.
62. Benbadis SR, Chichkova R. Psychogenic pseudosyncope: an underestimated and provable diagnosis. Epilepsy Behav. 2006;9:106–10.
63. Meadow R. Different interpretations of Munchausen syndrome by proxy. Child Abuse Negl. 2002;26:501–8.
64. Meadow R. What is, and what is not, 'Munchausen syndrome by proxy'? Arch Dis Child. 1995;72:534–8.
65. Schreier H. Munchausen by proxy defined. Pediatrics. 2002;110:985–8.
66. Thomas K. Munchausen syndrome by proxy: identification and diagnosis. J Pediatr Nurs. 2003;18:174–80.
67. Grady MM, Stahl SM. Panic attacks and panic disorders: the great imitators. In: Kaplan PW, Fisher RS, editors. Imitators of epilepsy. 2nd ed. New York: Demos; 2005. p. 277–88.
68. Sazgar M, Carlen PL, Wennberg R. Panic attack semiology in right temporal lobe epilepsy. Epileptic Disord. 2003;5:93–100.
69. varez-Silva S, varez-Rodriguez J, Perez-Echeverria MJ, varez-Silva I. Panic and epilepsy. J Anxiety Disord. 2006;20:353–62.
70. Evans RW. Neurologic aspects of hyperventilation syndrome. Semin Neurol. 1995;15:115–25.
71. Folgering H. The pathophysiology of hyperventilation syndrome. Monaldi Arch Chest Dis. 1999;54:365–72.
72. Baranes T, Rossignol B, Stheneur C, Bidat E. Hyperventilation syndrome in children. Arch Pediatr. 2005;12:1742–7.
73. Evans RW. Hyperventilation syndrome. In: Kaplan PW, Fisher RS, editors. Imitators of epilepsy. 2nd ed. New York: Demos; 2005. p. 241–53.
74. Lesser RP. Treatment and outcome of psychogenic nonepileptic seizures. Epilepsy Curr. 2003;3:198–200.
75. Reuber M, Howlett S, Kemp S. Psychologic treatment of patients with psychogenic nonepileptic seizures. Expert Rev Neurother. 2005;5:737–52.
76. Carton S, Thompson PJ, Duncan JS. Non-epileptic seizures: patients' understanding and reaction to the diagnosis and impact on outcome. Seizure. 2003;12:287–94.
77. Caviness JN, Brown P. Myoclonus: current concepts and recent advances. Lancet Neurol. 2004;3:598–607.
78. Vigevano F. Non-epileptic paroxysmal disorders in the first year of life. In: Panayiotopoulos CP, editor. A practical guide to childhood epilepsies, vol. 1. Oxford: Medicinae; 2006. p. 107–14.
79. Vigevano F, Lispi ML. Tonic reflex seizures of early infancy: an age-related non-epileptic paroxysmal disorder. Epileptic Disord. 2001;3:133–6.
80. Nechay A, Ross LM, Stephenson JB, O'regan M. Gratification disorder ("infantile masturbation"): a review. Arch Dis Child. 2004;89:225–6.
81. Daoust-Roy J, Seshia SS. Benign neonatal sleep myoclonus. A differential diagnosis of neonatal seizures. Am J Dis Child. 1992;146:1236–41.
82. Di Capua M, Fusco L, Ricci S, Vigevano F. Benign neonatal sleep myoclonus: clinical features and video-polygraphic recordings. Mov Disord. 1993;8:191–4.
83. Caraballo R, Yepez I, Cersosimo R, Fejerman N. Benign neonatal sleep myoclonus. Rev Neurol. 1998;26:540–4.
84. Pachatz C, Fusco L, Vigevano F. Benign myoclonus of early infancy. Epileptic Disord. 1999;1:57–61.
85. Kanazawa O. Shuddering attacks-report of four children. Pediatr Neurol. 2000;23:421–4.
86. Praveen V, Patole SK, Whitehall JS. Hyperekplexia in neonates. Postgrad Med J. 2001;77:570–2.
87. Bakker MJ, van Dijk JG, van den Maagdenberg AM, Tijssen MA. Startle syndromes. Lancet Neurol. 2006;5:513–24.
88. Cioni G, Biagioni E, Bottai P, Castellacci AM, Paolicelli PB. Hyperekplexia and stiff-baby syndrome: an identical neurological disorder? Ital J Neurol Sci. 1993;14:145–52.
89. Gomeza J, Ohno K, Hulsmann S, Armsen W, Eulenburg V, Richter DW, et al. Deletion of the mouse glycine transporter 2 results in a hyperekplexia phenotype and postnatal lethality. Neuron. 2003;40:797–806.
90. Castaldo P, Stefanoni P, Miceli F, Coppola G, del Giudice EM, Bellini G, et al. A novel hyperekplexia-causing mutation in the pre-transmembrane segment 1 of the human glycine receptor alpha1 subunit reduces membrane expression and impairs gating by agonists. J Biol Chem. 2004;279:25598–604.
91. Rees MI, Harvey K, Pearce BR, Chung SK, Duguid IC, Thomas P, et al. Mutations in the gene encoding GlyT2 (SLC6A5) define a presynaptic component of human startle disease 5. Nat Genet. 2006;38:801–6.

92. Brown P. Neurophysiology of the startle syndrome and hyperekplexia. Adv Neurol. 2002;89:153–9.
93. Ryan SG, Sherman SL, Terry JC, Sparkes RS, Torres MC, Mackey RW. Startle disease, or hyperekplexia: response to clonazepam and assignment of the gene (STHE) to chromosome 5q by linkage analysis. Ann Neurol. 1992;31:663–8.
94. Matsuo H, Kamakura K, Matsushita S, Ohmori T, Okano M, Tadano Y, et al. Mutational analysis of the anion exchanger 3 gene in familial paroxysmal dystonic choreoathetosis linked to chromosome 2q. Am J Med Genet. 1999;88:733–7.
95. Jarman PR, Bhatia KP, Davie C, Heales SJ, Turjanski N, Taylor-Robinson SD, et al. Paroxysmal dystonic choreoathetosis: clinical features and investigation of pathophysiology in a large family. Mov Disord. 2000;15:648–57.
96. Rainier S, Thomas D, Tokarz D, Ming L, Bui M, Plein E, et al. Myofibrillogenesis regulator 1 gene mutations cause paroxysmal dystonic choreoathetosis. Arch Neurol. 2004;61:1025–9.
97. Chatterjee A, Louis ED, Frucht S. Levetiracetam in the treatment of paroxysmal kinesiogenic choreoathetosis. Mov Disord. 2002;17:614–5.
98. Ohmori I, Ohtsuka Y, Ogino T, Yoshinaga H, Kobayashi K, Oka E. The relationship between paroxysmal kinesigenic choreoathetosis and epilepsy. Neuropediatrics. 2002;33:15–20.
99. Tsai JD, Chou IC, Tsai FJ, Kuo HT, Tsai CH. Clinical manifestation and carbamazepine treatment of patients with paroxysmal kinesigenic choreoathetosis. Acta Paediatr Taiwan. 2005;46:138–42.
100. Kato N, Sadamatsu M, Kikuchi T, Niikawa N, Fukuyama Y. Paroxysmal kinesigenic choreoathetosis: from first discovery in 1892 to genetic linkage with benign familial infantile convulsions. Epilepsy Res. 2006;70(Suppl):174–84.
101. Wein T, Andermann F, Silver K, Dubeau F, Andermann E, Rourke-Frew F, et al. Exquisite sensitivity of paroxysmal kinesigenic choreoathetosis to carbamazepine. Neurology. 1996;47:1104–6.
102. Hamada Y, Hattori H, Okuno T. Eleven cases of paroxysmal kinesigenic choreoathetosis; correlation with benign infantile convulsions. No To Hattatsu. 1998;30:483–8.
103. Kato N, Sadamatsu M, Kikuchi T, Niikawa N, Fukuyama Y. Paroxysmal kinesigenic choreoathetosis: from first discovery in 1892 to genetic linkage with benign familial infantile convulsions. Epilepsy Res. 2006;70(Suppl):174–84.
104. Escayg A, De Waard M, Lee DD, Bichet D, Wolf P, Mayer T, et al. Coding and noncoding variation of the human calcium-channel beta4-subunit gene CACNB4 in patients with idiopathic generalized epilepsy and episodic ataxia. Am J Hum Genet. 2000;66:1531–9.
105. Zuberi SM, Eunson LH, Spauschus A, De Silva R, Tolmie J, Wood NW, et al. A novel mutation in the human voltage-gated potassium channel gene (Kv1.1) associates with episodic ataxia type 1 and sometimes with partial epilepsy. Brain. 1999;122(Pt 5):817–25.
106. Imbrici P, D'Adamo MC, Cusimano A, Pessia M. Episodic ataxia type 1 mutation F184C alters Zn2+-induced modulation of the human potassium channel Kv1.4-Kv1.1/Kv{beta}1.1. Am J Physiol Cell Physiol. 2007;292:C778–87.
107. Eunson LH, Rea R, Zuberi SM, Youroukos S, Panayiotopoulos CP, Liguori R, et al. Clinical, genetic, and expression studies of mutations in the potassium channel gene KCNA1 reveal new phenotypic variability. Ann Neurol. 2000;48:647–56.
108. Palmini AL, Gloor P, Jones-Gotman M. Pure amnestic seizures in temporal lobe epilepsy. Definition, clinical symptomatology and functional anatomical considerations. Brain. 1992;115(Pt 3):749–69.
109. Sander K, Sander D. New insights into transient global amnesia: recent imaging and clinical findings. Lancet Neurol. 2005;4:437–44.
110. Quinette P, Guillery-Girard B, Dayan J, de La Sayette V, Marquis S, Viader F, et al. What does transient global amnesia really mean? Review of the literature and thorough study of 142 cases. Brain. 2006;129(Pt 7):1640–58.
111. Kopelman MD, Panayiotopoulos CP, Lewis P. Transient epileptic amnesia differentiated from psychogenic "fugue": neuropsychological, EEG, and PET findings. J Neurol Neurosurg Psychiatr. 1994;57:1002–4.
112. Cascino GD. Clinical indications and diagnostic yield of video-electroencephalographic monitoring in patients with seizures and spells. Mayo Clin Proc. 2002;77:1111–20.
113. Rosenow F, Wyllie E, Kotagal P, Mascha E, Wolgamuth BR, Hamer H. Staring spells in children: descriptive features distinguishing epileptic and nonepileptic events. J Pediatr. 1998;133:660–3.
114. Ferrie CD. Non-convulsive attacks imitating epileptic seizures (non-epileptic absences). In: Panayiotopoulos CP, editor. A practical guide to childhood epilepsies, vol. 1. Oxford: Medicinae; 2006. p. 139–43.
115. Kotagal P, Costa M, Wyllie E, Wolgamuth B. Paroxysmal nonepileptic events in children and adolescents. Pediatrics. 2002;110:e46.
116. Roberts R. Differential diagnosis of sleep disorders, non-epileptic attacks and epileptic seizures. Curr Opin Neurol. 1998;11:135–9.
117. Kotagal S. Parasomnias in childhood. Sleep Med Rev. 2009;13:157–68.
118. Stores G. Aspects of parasomnias in childhood and adolescence. Arch Dis Child. 2009;94:63–9.
119. Bazil CW. Parasomnias, sleep disorders and narcolepsy – sleep-time imitators of epilepsy. In: Kaplan PW, Fisher RS, editors. Imitators of epilepsy. 2nd ed. New York: Demos; 2005. p. 217–30.

120. Mason TB, Pack AI. Pediatric parasomnias. Sleep. 2007;30:141–51.
121. Avidan AY. Parasomnias and movement disorders of sleep. Semin Neurol. 2009;29:372–92.
122. Pressman MR. Factors that predispose, prime and precipitate NREM parasomnias in adults: clinical and forensic implications. Sleep Med Rev. 2007;11:5–30.
123. Gowers WR. The borderland of epilepsy: faints, vagal attacks, vertigo, migraine, sleep symptoms, and their treatment. Philadelphia: P. Blakiston's Son & Co.; 1907.
124. Dinner DS. Sleep and pediatric epilepsy. Cleve Clin J Med. 1989;56(Suppl Pt 2):S234–9.
125. Bourgeois B. The relationship between sleep and epilepsy in children. Semin Pediatr Neurol. 1996;3:29–35.
126. Autret A, Lucas B, Hommet C, Corcia P, de Toffol B. Sleep and the epilepsies. J Neurol. 1997; 244(Suppl):S10–7.
127. Crespel A, Coubes P, Baldy-Moulinier M. Sleep influence on seizures and epilepsy effects on sleep in partial frontal and temporal lobe epilepsies. Clin Neurophysiol. 2000;111 Suppl 2:S54–9.
128. Bazil CW. Sleep-related epilepsy. Curr Neurol Neurosci Rep. 2003;3:167–72.
129. Bazil CW. Effects of antiepileptic drugs on sleep structure: are all drugs equal? CNS Drugs. 2003;17: 719–28.
130. D'Alessandro R, Guarino M, Greco G, Bassein L. Risk of seizures while awake in pure sleep epilepsies: a prospective study. Neurology. 2004;62:254–7.
131. Schenck CH, Mahowald MW. Parasomnias. Managing bizarre sleep-related behavior disorders. Postgrad Med. 2000;107:145–56.
132. American Sleep Disorders Association. International classification of sleep disorders: diagnostic and coding manual. Rochester: American Sleep Disorders Association; 1990.
133. Oswald I. Sudden bodily jerks on falling asleep. Brain. 1959;82:92–103.
134. Bixler EO, Kales A, Vela-Bueno A, Jacoby JA, Scarone S, Soldatos CR. Nocturnal myoclonus and nocturnal myoclonic activity in the normal population. Res Commun Chem Pathol Pharmacol. 1982;36: 129–40.
135. Broughton R, Tolentino MA, Krelina M. Excessive fragmentary myoclonus in NREM sleep: a report of 38 cases. Electroencephalogr Clin Neurophysiol. 1985;61:123–33.
136. Lins O, Castonguay M, Dunham W, Nevsimalova S, Broughton R. Excessive fragmentary myoclonus: time of night and sleep stage distributions. Can J Neurol Sci. 1993;20:142–6.
137. Vetrugno R, Plazzi G, Provini F, Liguori R, Lugaresi E, Montagna P. Excessive fragmentary hypnic myoclonus: clinical and neurophysiological findings. Sleep Med. 2002;3:73–6.
138. Montagna P, Provini F, Plazzi G, Liguori R, Lugaresi E. Propriospinal myoclonus upon relaxation and drowsiness: a cause of severe insomnia. Mov Disord. 1997;12:66–72.
139. Vetrugno R, Provini F, Meletti S, Plazzi G, Liguori R, Cortelli P, et al. Propriospinal myoclonus at the sleep-wake transition: a new type of parasomnia. Sleep. 2001;24:835–43.
140. Vetrugno R, Provini F, Plazzi G, Cortelli P, Montagna P. Propriospinal myoclonus: a motor phenomenon found in restless legs syndrome different from periodic limb movements during sleep. Mov Disord. 2005;20:1323–9.
141. Vetrugno R, Provini F, Plazzi G, Lombardi C, Liguori R, Lugaresi E, et al. Familial nocturnal faciomandibular myoclonus mimicking sleep bruxism. Neurology. 2002;58:644–7.
142. Lesage S, Hening WA. The restless legs syndrome and periodic limb movement disorder: a review of management. Semin Neurol. 2004;24:249–59.
143. Carrier J, Frenette S, Montplaisir J, Paquet J, Drapeau C, Morettini J. Effects of periodic leg movements during sleep in middle-aged subjects without sleep complaints. Mov Disord. 2005;20:1127–32.
144. Ferri R, Zucconi M, Manconi M, Plazzi G, Bruni O, Ferini-Strambi L. New approaches to the study of periodic leg movements during sleep in restless legs syndrome. Sleep. 2006;29:759–69.
145. Zucconi M, Ferri R, Allen R, Baier PC, Bruni O, Chokroverty S, et al. The official World Association of Sleep Medicine (WASM) standards for recording and scoring periodic leg movements in sleep (PLMS) and wakefulness (PLMW) developed in collaboration with a task force from the International Restless Legs Syndrome Study Group (IRLSSG). Sleep Med. 2006;7:175–83.
146. Wetter TC, Pollmacher T. Restless legs and periodic leg movements in sleep syndromes. J Neurol. 1997;244 Suppl 1:S37–45.
147. Mahowald MW. Restless leg syndrome and periodic limb movements of sleep. Curr Treat Options Neurol. 2003;5:251–60.
148. Szelenberger W, Niemcewicz S, Dabrowska AJ. Sleepwalking and night terrors: psychopathological and psychophysiological correlates. Int Rev Psychiatry. 2005;17:263–70.
149. Guilleminault C, Palombini L, Pelayo R, Chervin RD. Sleepwalking and sleep terrors in prepubertal children: what triggers them? Pediatrics. 2003;111:e17–25.
150. Amir N, Navon P, Silverberg-Shalev R. Interictal electroencephalography in night terrors and somnambulism. Isr J Med Sci. 1985;21:22–6.
151. Roth B, Nevsimalova S, Sagova V, Paroubkova D, Horakova A. Neurological, psychological and polygraphic findings in sleep drunkenness. Schweiz Arch Neurol Neurochir Psychiatr. 1981;129:209–22.

152. Mahowald MW, Schenck CH. Dissociated states of wakefulness and sleep. Neurology. 1992;42 Suppl 6:44–51.
153. Clark GT, Ram S. Four oral motor disorders: bruxism, dystonia, dyskinesia and drug-induced dystonic extrapyramidal reactions. Dent Clin North Am. 2007;51:225–43.
154. Herrera M, Valencia I, Grant M, Metroka D, Chialastri A, Kothare SV. Bruxism in children: effect on sleep architecture and daytime cognitive performance and behavior. Sleep. 2006;29:1143–8.
155. Lobbezoo F, Van Der ZJ, Naeije M. Bruxism: its multiple causes and its effects on dental implants - an updated review. J Oral Rehabil. 2006;33:293–300.
156. Winocur E, Hermesh H, Littner D, Shiloh R, Peleg L, Eli I. Signs of bruxism and temporomandibular disorders among psychiatric patients. Oral Surg Oral Med Oral Pathol Oral Radiol Endod. 2007;103: 60–3.
157. Vetrugno R, Provini F, Plazzi G, Vignatelli L, Lugaresi E, Montagna P. Catathrenia (nocturnal groaning): a new type of parasomnia. Neurology. 2001;56:681–3.
158. Makari J, Rushton HG. Nocturnal enuresis. Am Fam Physician. 2006;73:1611–3.
159. Olson EJ, Boeve BF, Silber MH. Rapid eye movement sleep behaviour disorder: demographic, clinical and laboratory findings in 93 cases. Brain. 2000;123(Pt 2):331–9.
160. Fantini ML, Corona A, Clerici S, Ferini-Strambi L. Aggressive dream content without daytime aggressiveness in REM sleep behavior disorder. Neurology. 2005;65:1010–5.
161. Fantini ML, Ferini-Strambi L, Montplaisir J. Idiopathic REM sleep behavior disorder: toward a better nosologic definition. Neurology. 2005;64:780–6.
162. Gagnon JF, Postuma RB, Montplaisir J. Update on the pharmacology of REM sleep behavior disorder. Neurology. 2006;67:742–7.
163. Thirumalai SS, Shubin RA, Robinson R. Rapid eye movement sleep behavior disorder in children with autism. J Child Neurol. 2002;17:173–8.
164. Manni R, Terzaghi M, Zambrelli E, Pacchetti C. Interictal, potentially misleading, epileptiform EEG abnormalities in REM sleep behavior disorder. Sleep. 2006;29:934–7.
165. Vetrugno R, Manconi M, Ferini-Strambi L, Provini F, Plazzi G, Montagna P. Nocturnal eating: sleep-related eating disorder or night eating syndrome? A videopolysomnographic study. Sleep. 2006;29: 949–54.
166. Kinney HC, Thach BT. The sudden infant death syndrome. N Engl J Med. 2009;361:795–805.
167. Billiard M, Bassetti C, Dauvilliers Y, Dolenc-Groselj L, Lammers GJ, Mayer G, et al. EFNS guidelines on management of narcolepsy. Eur J Neurol. 2006;13:1035–48.
168. Dauvilliers Y, Tafti M. Molecular genetics and treatment of narcolepsy. Ann Med. 2006;38:252–62.
169. Erman MK. Selected sleep disorders: restless legs syndrome and periodic limb movement disorder, sleep apnea syndrome, and narcolepsy. Psychiatr Clin North Am. 2006;29:947–67.
170. Kawashima M, Tamiya G, Oka A, Hohjoh H, Juji T, Ebisawa T, et al. Genomewide association analysis of human narcolepsy and a new resistance gene. Am J Hum Genet. 2006;79:252–63.
171. Mazzetti M, Campi C, Mattarozzi K, Plazzi G, Tuozzi G, Vandi S, et al. Semantic priming effect during REM-sleep inertia in patients with narcolepsy. Brain Res Bull. 2006;71:270–8.
172. Siegel JM, Boehmer LN. Narcolepsy and the hypocretin system – where motion meets emotion. Nat Clin Pract Neurol. 2006;2:548–56.
173. Stores G. The protean manifestations of childhood narcolepsy and their misinterpretation. Dev Med Child Neurol. 2006;48:307–10.
174. Thorpy MJ. Cataplexy associated with narcolepsy: epidemiology, pathophysiology and management. CNS Drugs. 2006;20:43–50.
175. Wurtman RJ. Narcolepsy and the hypocretins. Metabolism. 2006;55 Suppl 2:S36–9.
176. Feinsilver SH. Sleep in the elderly. What is normal? Clin Geriatr Med. 2003;19:177–88, viii.
177. Mazza M, Della MG, De RS, Mennuni GF, Mazza S. Sleep disorders in the elderly. Clin Ter. 2004; 155:391–4.
178. FineSmith R, Geller EB, Devinsky O. Strange tastes, smell, sounds, visions and feelings: nonepileptic events that mimic simple partial seizures. In: Kaplan PW, Fisher RS, editors. Imitators of epilepsy. 2nd ed. New York: Demos; 2005. p. 133–43.
179. Critchley M. Types of visual perseveration: 'palinopsia' and 'illusory visual spread'. Brain. 1951;74:267–99.
180. Spanos NP, Stam HJ. The elicitation of visual hallucinations via brief instructions in a normal sample. J Nerv Ment Dis. 1979;167:488–94.
181. Kolmel HW. Visual illusions and hallucinations. Baillieres Clin Neurol. 1993;2:243–64.
182. Manford M, Andermann F. Complex visual hallucinations. Clinical and neurobiological insights. Brain. 1998;121(Pt 10):1819–40.
183. Wilkinson F. Auras and other hallucinations: windows on the visual brain. Prog Brain Res. 2004;144:305–20.
184. Panayiotopoulos CP. Panayiotopoulos syndrome: a common and benign childhood epileptic syndrome. London: John Libbey & Co. Ltd; 2002.

185. Li BU, Balint JP. Cyclic vomiting syndrome: evolution in our understanding of a brain-gut disorder. Adv Pediatr. 2000;47:117–60.
186. Li BU, Issenman RM, Sarna SK. Consensus statement – 2nd international scientific symposium on CVS. The faculty of the 2nd international scientific symposium on cyclic vomiting syndrome. Dig Dis Sci. 1999;44(Suppl):9S–11.
187. Andrews PL. Cyclic vomiting syndrome: timing, targets, and treatment – a basic science perspective. Dig Dis Sci. 1999;44(Suppl):31S–8.
188. Zajonc TP, Roland PS. Vertigo and motion sickness. Part I: vestibular anatomy and physiology. Ear Nose Throat J. 2005;84:581–4.
189. Bosser G, Caillet G, Gauchard G, Marcon F, Perrin P. Relation between motion sickness susceptibility and vasovagal syncope susceptibility. Brain Res Bull. 2006;68:217–26.
190. Golding JF. Motion sickness susceptibility. Auton Neurosci. 2006;129:67–76.
191. Shupak A, Gordon CR. Motion sickness: advances in pathogenesis, prediction, prevention, and treatment. Aviat Space Environ Med. 2006;77:1213–23.
192. Zajonc TP, Roland PS. Vertigo and motion sickness. Part II: pharmacologic treatment. Ear Nose Throat J. 2006;85:25–35.
193. Panayiotopoulos CP. Differentiating occipital epilepsies from migraine with aura, acephalgic migraine and basilar migraine. In: Panayiotopoulos CP, editor. Benign childhood partial seizures and related epileptic syndromes. London: John Libbey & Co. Ltd; 1999. p. 281–302.
194. Panayiotopoulos CP. Elementary visual hallucinations, blindness, and headache in idiopathic occipital epilepsy: differentiation from migraine. J Neurol Neurosurg Psychiatry. 1999;66:536–40.
195. Panayiotopoulos CP. Visual phenomena and headache in occipital epilepsy: a review, a systematic study and differentiation from migraine. Epileptic Disord. 1999;1:205–16.
196. Panayiotopoulos CP. "Migralepsy" and the significance of differentiating occipital seizures from migraine. Epilepsia. 2006;47:806–8.
197. Herschel JFW. Familiar lectures on scientific aspects. London: Alexander Straham; 1866.
198. Russell MB, Olesen J. A nosographic analysis of the migraine aura in a general population. Brain. 1996; 119(Pt 2):355–61.
199. Bickerstaff ER. Basilar artery migraine. Lancet. 1961;i:15–7.
200. Bickerstaff ER. Impairment of consciousness in migraine. Lancet. 1961;ii:1057–9.
201. Panayiotopoulos CP. Basilar migraine: a review. In: Panayiotopoulos CP, editor. Benign childhood partial seizures and related epileptic syndromes. London: John Libbey & Co. Ltd; 1999. p. 303–8.
202. Lennox WG, Lennox MA. Epilepsy and related disorders. Boston: Little, Brown & Co.; 1960.
203. Marks DA, Ehrenberg BL. Migraine-related seizures in adults with epilepsy, with EEG correlation. Neurology. 1993;43:2476–83.
204. Terzano MG, Parrino L, Pietrini V, Galli L. Migraine-epilepsy syndrome:intercalated seizures in benign occipital epilepsy. In: Andermann F, Beaumanoir A, Mira L, Roger J, Tassinari CA, editors. Occipital seizures and epilepsies in children. London: John Libbey & Co. Ltd; 1993. p. 93–9.
205. Slatter KH. Some clinical and EEG findings in patients with migraine. Brain. 1968;91:85–98.
206. Barlow CF. Headaches and migraine in childhood. Oxford: Blackwell Scientific Publications Ltd; 1984.
207. Holmes G. Sabill memorial oration on focal epilepsy. Lancet. 1927;i:957–62.
208. Panayiotopoulos CP. Elementary visual hallucinations in migraine and epilepsy. J Neurol Neurosurg Psychiatry. 1994;57:1371–4.
209. Camfield PR, Metrakos K, Andermann F. Basilar migraine, seizures, and severe epileptiform EEG abnormalities. Neurology. 1978;28:584–8.
210. Panayiotopoulos CP. Basilar migraine? Seizures, and severe epileptic EEG abnormalities. Neurology. 1980;30:1122–5.
211. De Romanis F, Buzzi MG, Assenza S, Brusa L, Cerbo R. Basilar migraine with electroencephalographic findings of occipital spike-wave complexes: a long-term study in seven children. Cephalalgia. 1993;13: 192–6.
212. Panayiotopoulos CP. Basilar migraine. Neurology. 1991;41:1707.
213. Ludvigsson P, Hesdorffer D, Olafsson E, Kjartansson O, Hauser WA. Migraine with aura is a risk factor for unprovoked seizures in children. Ann Neurol. 2006;59:210–3.
214. Commission of Classification and Terminology of the International League Against Epilepsy. Proposal for revised clinical and electroencephalographic classification of epileptic seizures. Epilepsia 1981;22:489–501.
215. Engel J Jr. Report of the ILAE Classification Core Group. Epilepsia 2006;47:1558–68.

Index

C.P. Panayiotopoulos, *Imitators of Epileptic Seizures*,
DOI 10.1007/ 978-1-4471-4023-8, © Springer-Verlag London 2012